PUBLISHING

LEAN STONE PUBLISHING

"Turn the Page And Live a Better Life"

www.leanstonebookclub.com

Health, Bundle I
Fertility, Intermittent Fasting

Table of Contents

Fertility

How to Get Pregnant – Cure Infertility, Get Pregnant & Start Expecting a Baby

Introduction

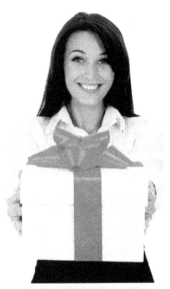
Seeking to get pregnant? Then, you've reached the right place. Determining to have a baby is, probably, the most important decision you will make in your life. But what if you know you

are ready to become a parent, but still, nothing happens? You know how you deeply yearn to become a mother, but you have been diagnosed with infertility.

Through this book, I want to show you that there are things you can consider, which you haven't tried yet, that will make your dream come true. I want you to concentrate on understanding your body. If you're getting impatient and the victim of negativity, don't let that get to you. Bear this in mind, your emotions can significantly influence the way in which your body functions, so my very first piece of advice would be to try to be as positive as possible and open-minded. If you're attempting to get pregnant and it seems like the odds are against you, then you shouldn't despair, there is a myriad of things for you to do, which can help you increase your chances of growing a baby inside of you.

For starters, understanding how pregnancy happens is crucial. That is one of the first aspects we're going to deal with in this book. If you have a lot of questions on your mind concerning the process of getting pregnant, essential tips on how to increase your chances of achieving that, and curing infertility, this book is perfect for you. It will help you comprehend the most important aspects related to pregnancy and understand what prevents you from getting pregnant. So, by the time you will have finished reading this book, you will indeed be filled with useful knowledge on the subject!

Also, you need to understand how your body works. If there are certain habits in your daily lifestyle that, without your knowledge, may be lowering your chances of expecting a baby. Sometimes, a broad range of habits or little customs can be harmful, and we might not even know it. There is evidence indicating that certain practices can significantly affect the body and decrease its fertility. Lack of knowledge can restrain your chances; that's a given. The human body is complex, and there might be aspects that you're unaware of. That's why being always informed is a positive idea. And we'll get into that in the following chapters.

Nothing equals the feeling of expecting a baby, and knowing that after a long period of wait, that little, tiny person in your arms is yours forever! Everyone dreams about that precious moment, why not admit it? Because no family is complete without the loveliness that a child brings once he/she enters the world. And when that happens, we feel like our world would be empty without that little person. It will happen to you, as well.

Without further ado, let's delve into this abundant subject. We'll get every little thing clarified. I truly want you to comprehend the process of getting pregnant while explaining the most important thing related to the subject that you might have heard and might have discouraged you immensely. This book encompasses all you need to know so that you can start expecting your baby soon. Good luck!

Chapter 1: Understand the Process of Getting Pregnant

In this chapter, you will learn:

- What the process of getting pregnant involves
- How your body functions
- Basic tips on how to improve your chances of getting pregnant

Let's cut it down to the chase. Even though most of us are quite curious about the mysterious act of conception, the greater majority of us don't comprehend how intriguing this process really is. But, curious or not, if you're looking to get pregnant, it's vital that you grasp the complicated process.

One of the fundamental pieces of advice for women who are trying to get pregnant is to get to know their bodies, more exactly, their menstrual cycle. Additionally, equally important is to comprehend how pregnancy takes place. You need to find out what happens inside your body. Believe me, it can make all the difference in the world!

First of all, how does pregnancy begin? The process of getting pregnant starts with the release of the egg from the ovary. This process is called ovulation. Afterward, the fertile egg must encounter the sperm, and form a particular cell; this step is known as fertilization. Next, this individual cell must reach the uterus of the woman and start developing. That is implementation. Now, the cell begins to grow and keep on growing until it becomes a human being. It makes sense, right?

What happens during ovulation?

Women are born with a large number of immature eggs, up to millions. However, only hundreds will mature. Typically, an egg is about the size of a pinhead.

Normally, the average menstrual cycle is between 28 and 32 days. For younger women, the menstrual cycle may last up to 45 days. Ovulation takes place somewhere between day 11 and 21 of your cycle, depending on its length and regularity. The luteinizing hormone prepares the release of the egg from the ovary. During this time, your cervical mucus has to be increasingly more slippery and thinner in consistency.

The greater majority of women experience slight aches during ovulation, so this might be a sign showing that you're ovulating. Also, ovulation changes your body's temperature. This is why some women measure their bodies' temperature in order to detect the peak of their fertility. In some cases, ovulation equals in a growth in sex drive.

Now, the egg released by the ovaries travels through the fallopian tubes. This action occurs one time per cycle. In some cases, two or even more eggs are released, and in case they are both fertilized, there can be a case of twins or even triplets.

Typically, the fallopian tubes are the spot where fertilization takes place. Every ovary is linked to a fallopian tube. Inside the fallopian tubes, there are small pieces of hair known as cilia. They facilitate the passing through process of the egg from the ovary to the uterus. The entire course lasts for several days during which the egg is perfectly preserved and nourished.

All this time, the uterus has developed an internal lining known as endometrium that is filled with nutrients that will protect and nurture the egg once it reaches the uterus. However, if the egg isn't fertilized, it disintegrates into the endometrium, which will be released during your monthly period.

What are the chances of conceiving twins or triplets?

That is a question I hear on a regular basis. First, how often does this happen, and secondly – is there something one can do for increasing the likelihood of conceiving twins and triplets? Find out that, in recent years, there has been a significant increase in multiple births. In fact, ever since 1980, the rate of triplet births is five times higher than in the previous years. In 2000 alone, in the United States, the following birth statistics were recorded:

- 118,920 twin births

- 6,740 triplet births

- 507 quadruplet births

- 78 quintuplets and other multiple births

These statics indicate that, compared to the past, there has been an increase of 70 percent in multiple births. The year 2000 has recorded 4 billion births in the States, and 3 percent of the total was multiple births. While conceiving triplets isn't an ordinary happening, it's a possibility.

What are your chances of having more than one baby at a time?

Typically speaking, it all comes down to this – 3 percent, or one in thirty-three births. The likelihood of conceiving "natural" fraternal twins is one in sixty – 1.7 percent – while the odds of having identical twins have remained still, being of 0.4 percent, namely one in two hundred fifty cases. However, by choosing to opt for fertility treatments, mothers can improve these odds and make them as high as 25 percent.

Ok, now that we've settled that, let's move on to the next commonly met question – what factors are recognized as responsible for increasing these odds?

Fertility medicine

It appears that the intake of fertility medicine is the first factor that will weigh the balance towards aiding you to conceive twins or triplets. Being in line with the statistics, these drugs increase the likelihood as much as 25 percent.

Family history

The next on the list is your family history. In other words, if your mother and your grandmother have had multiple births, this will considerably enhance your odds of being pregnant with twins or triplets.

Previous pregnancies

According to statistics, women who have been pregnant in the past with more than two or three pregnancies present higher chances of conceiving twins or triplets.

Age

Another deciding factor is the mother's age. It appears that a woman's chances of conceiving twins increase as she ages. In fact, for women aged between 30 and 34, the likelihood increases with about 4 percent. For women above 35 years old, the probability further rises with another 5 percent.

Cultural background

As odd as it appears, it's interesting to note that the cultural context is an aspect that is critical in multiple births as well. It would seem that African Americans are more likely to deliver multiple babies while Hispanic and Asian women present the lowest rates in multiple births.

The fertilization process

As long as the sperm remains inside the fallopian tubes, it's able to fertilize the egg. However, if the fallopian tubes hold no egg inside, you are unable to conceive.

The fallopian tubes are 10 centimeters long, and they aim at delivering the egg from the ovary and afterward to the uterus. They also nourish the egg and the sperm to facilitate the perfect conceiving environment.

Typically, eggs are prone to remain in the tubes for about a day after being released. If they're not fertilized, they'll disintegrate. This particular day is the perfect timing for a woman to conceive. Sometimes, fertilization can occur even if the sexual intercourse happened days before the release of the egg. That is because the sperm can survive inside the tubes for a couple of days.

When the egg enters the tube, sperm cells become more active as they can sense the presence of the egg because of progesterone. Progesterone is a peculiar smell released by the egg. But how does the sperm manage to penetrate the egg? The moment when the head of the sperm encounters the egg, it will release particular enzymes that will enable its passing through. After the sperm enters the egg, we can say that fertilization has taken place. Right now, the fetus' DNA is set in stone.

The moment the sperm has fertilized the egg, the egg receives a protective cover that prevents other sperm from entering.

To conceive, you need to settle the peak fertility point of your menstrual cycle, which is the ovulation and the perfect timing for you and your partner to try to conceive. If you've been attempting to get pregnant without taking into consideration your ovulation peak, then the odds are you didn't succeed. Doctors say that a lot of couples fail to pay attention to this "tiny" detail and end up being disappointed. The following tips are useful in helping you understand when you're ovulating.

#1 Record menstrual cycle on a regular basis

Now, you need to record your menstrual cycle, so that you know what time of the month your body is fertile so that you can get pregnant. You need to pay attention whether your period comes the same time of the month regularly. Consider noting the dates of your periods on a calendar. If you notice that your cycle times and lengths vary from month to month, then you might have irregular periods, which can be the primary factor preventing you from conceiving. That is the first step when trying to conceive, record your menstrual cycles, and indicate when your ovary releases the egg.

Keep in mind that after the egg is released from the ovary, it is only fertile for 24 up to 48 hours tops. On the other hand, a man's sperm will remain in the woman's body untouched for up to six days. This is why you need to spot the moment when your body is ovulating.

If you're having trouble recording your menstrual cycle, one of the common causes of irregular periods is that birth control methods tend to disrupt the way in which your body normally functions. Thus, it will probably take a while until your menstrual cycles get back on track and become regular. Sometimes, it could take up to three months for women who used oral contraceptives to get regular menstrual periods. Don't worry; a lot of women have experienced this.

#2 Monitor ovulation

Most women who have regular menstrual cycles ovulate appreciatively two weeks before the date of the next period. Now, women who deal with irregular menstrual cycles may find this task rather difficult, but as a general pointer, ovulation happens 12 up to 16 days before the next period.

But, is there something you can do so that you monitor ovulation effectively? Yes. There are home ovulation prediction kits that can be helpful in determining when you're ovulating. A lot of women claim that these packages are extremely useful for this purpose, and doctors, in particular, recommend them. You could give them a try if you have problems monitoring your ovulation. You can find these kits in the majority of drug stores. A regular kit includes urine tests that determine the presence of luteinizing hormone, which is a substance whose levels typically grow in the ovulation period. As a general pointer, three days after a positive test result is, possibly, the right timing to try to conceive, as your chances of getting fertilized are certainly higher. Now, here's a list of the main pros and cons of using these ovulation kits, so that you can make an informed decision.

Pros of ovulation kits

[16]

Compared to other methods of monitoring ovulation, these kits are recognized as the most reliable. When they're used correctly, in more than 97 percent of the cases, the result is accurate.

They are convenient. Typically, you should use this type of kit in the middle of your cycle, when ovulation is most likely to occur. Alternatively, other methods require a daily commitment and a significant amount of time.

They are widely available. As previously mentioned, you can get this type of kit in any drugstore or supermarket.

They are easy to use. They operate directly, similarly to pregnancy tests. After urinating on the stick, it should indicate the LH surge, and give you a clear indicator concerning your ovulation. Most kits consist of five to nine sticks, depending on the price range as well.

Cons of ovulation kits

They don't test ovulation per say. This procedure aims at measuring the LH surge, which precedes ovulation. However, it cannot confirm or infirm that you have ovulated or not. There are cases in which an egg may fail to form, even after the LH surge has emerged – this condition is referred to as LUFS – luteinized unruptured follicle syndrome.

These kits don't point whether the cervical mucus is favorable for fertilization or not. The mucus that your body produces in the middle of the ovulation period is expected to present a particular consistency – it should be white and clear, such as egg whites. An ovulation kit doesn't monitor the cervical mucus. Alternatively, upon using the kit, you should aim at keeping track of your cervical mucus as well.

They don't work if you are on a type of fertility treatment. When you're administrating fertility medicine, the results shown by the kit cannot be trusted.

They don't show consistent results for women over 40. For women who are approaching their menopause phase, typically, those over 40, the levels of LH in their systems are usually higher. Hence the tests may be invalid and untrusted.

They aren't exactly cheap. Such a kit costs between $15 and $50, depending on the number of sticks included and the brand. You should purchase one for every cycle.

It is best to use such an ovulation kit, while aiming at keeping track of other indicators your body is giving you. For instance, another clear indicator of your ovulation period is your body's temperature. Believe it or not, your body's temperature reflects when you're ovulating. It's weird, I know, but that's the way it is. As a matter of fact, after ovulation, a woman's basal body temperature increases with less than half a degree Fahrenheit, or 0.3 degree Celsius. A woman's fertility reaches its peak during the two or three days before this growth in body temperature.

You can also depict your ovulation by carefully monitoring your cervical mucus. More precisely, monitoring your cervical mucus means paying close attention to the amount and appearance of the mucus. As you reach ovulation, the amount of cervical mucus significantly increases. Also, its consistency slightly alters as well – as it becomes clear and slippery. This will aid the sperm to reach the egg in less time, and fertilize it more quickly.

#3 The perfect timing

After figuring your fertile days, it's time you try to conceive your baby during your most fertile days. More exactly, three days before your ovulation period until the peak of your fertility. Starting a little sooner won't hurt anyone, won't it? As a matter of fact, some women I know have gotten pregnant six days before they were ovulating. As I already mentioned, the sperm remains in the woman's body for up to six days. Given this fact, it is best to opt for trying to conceive a few days before your ovulation (and keep "working" on that until menstruation) as the lifespan of the egg is 24 to 48 hours while the sperm survives increasingly more. To be clearer, if you attempt to conceive on Monday, the sperm is most likely to survive in your fallopian tubes waiting for the egg to come until Friday, even Saturday.

If you're not that confident concerning your ovulation time, because of your irregular menstrual cycles, at least, try to spot the approximate time of your ovulation by trying one of the methods I've mentioned before, and try to conceive daily in the proximity of that assumed time. If your fallopian tubes have the sperm waiting for an egg to float, as the sperm can survive up to 6 days, you'll increase your odds of getting pregnant soon.

Do irregular menstrual cycles make it harder to get pregnant?

Typically, irregular menstrual cycles can occur because of a range of factors including birth control intake for a considerable amount of time, dietary and lifestyle habits, health conditions such as thyroid disorders or polycystic ovarian syndrome. If you suffer from these health conditions, they could be the main factors deterring you from conceiving. Irregular or abnormal ovulation is estimated to be the cause of infertility in 30 percent of the cases.

It is recommendable to settle the reason you have irregular periods. After you have given up birth control for a while and you have implemented a couple of lifestyle changes we are going to discuss later, your menstrual cycle should be back on track. The fact is that your menstrual cycle is the result of a myriad of health and environmental factors, which means that an unhealthy lifestyle, with a lot of stress, and bad eating habits, or anorexia, all these can cause your ovulation to be irregular.

The more irregular your cycles are, the more difficult it is for you to monitor them, and find out when you're ovulating.

Because, when you're trying to have a baby, timing plays such an important role, you truly need to depict when your body reaches its fertility peak. From my personal experience, the disturbance of having irregular menstrual cycles can be solved by implementing a range of dietary and lifestyle changes. The tips I enumerated above can also aid you to notice when your body is ready to have a baby. Monitoring your body temperature or your cervical mucus, these can help you spot that one moment of the month that will make it possible for you to conceive.

Some women dealing with irregular cycles can keep track of them by using ovulation prediction kits.

When should I worry?

I would say it's never best for you to start worrying. Did you know that stressed couples are 30 percent less likely to conceive? Still, most couples who haven't gotten pregnant right away seem to be quite stressed about it. You need to understand that it depends on each couple and their environmental and lifestyle choices. When it takes too long to conceive, couples tend to get worried and assume the worst, and these negative feelings and frustration are making it worse, believe me.

To some extent, it is a very natural concern, to worry when you have tried to get pregnant for a while now and did not succeed. In our fast-paced, modern world, we wish to be given what we want right away, and we tend to become overly frustrated in cases of infertility. Think about it, you get a processed meal from the supermarket and cook it in less than 15 minutes. You can fly across the continent for a couple of hours. As responsible and as in control as we may seem to be when it comes to getting pregnant, you have to listen to your body. Sometimes, your body needs to be properly taken care of before it has the right foundation for carrying a pregnancy.

Still, I heartedly advise you don't overlook these worries and emotions and consider scheduling some time with a physician to talk about your case. In some circumstances, the reassurance from specialists is all it takes for some couples to get pregnant. You shouldn't compare your situation with that of another couple because everyone presents its individual set of features.

Chapter 2: Common Causes of Infertility in both Men and Women

In this chapter, you will learn:

- The most common causes of infertility in women and men
- The primary symptoms associated with these conditions
- The various treatment options for infertility
- The latest research on the topic

About eleven percent of the couples trying to conceive in the United States encounter difficulties. In one-third of the cases, the root of the problem is female infertility, in one-third we're talking about male infertility and the rest is typically caused by a mixture of unexplained factors. The good news is that more than 65 percent of the couples that deal with these issues can conceive successfully.

Unfortunately, life isn't fair. We find this out every day as bad things happen to us, and we are unable to control them. Life isn't fair when your rude colleague gets promoted instead of you. But, most of all, life's unfair when you try to get pregnant, and, somehow, that becomes impossible because of infertility. Nothing is more stressing than attempting to conceive and experiencing a mixture of negative feelings and guilt, because, somehow, your body is unable to accomplish that.

But that's just life, women who don't plan on getting pregnant, somehow, they do, and those who yearn to become mothers are endlessly trying with no success.

I know that all these thoughts are always tormenting you because it's tough to be a yearning mother with no child. But, you have to let go of all these negative feelings and anger that you might be experiencing – whether you're directing it towards yourself or your partner, it's harming you more than you know it. I will expand on this matter a little bit later throughout the book. But right now, I want to present to you the most common causes of infertility in women and men.

Ovulation problems

An ovulation problem frequently refers to the situation in which the eggs don't develop in the ovaries or the ovaries are unable to release a healthy egg. These are quite common. Symptoms are infrequent or absent menstrual cycles, inexistent or heavy menstrual bleeding.

In some cases, ovulation problems can be fixed with a few lifestyle changes such as a healthy body weight, a proper diet and, taking the necessary supplements.

Endometriosis

As you already read above, the woman's body is preparing for conceiving on a monthly basis. The lining attached to the uterus – the endometrium – thickens and is filled with red blood cells. Afterward, the ovaries release the egg. If the sperm doesn't fertilize the egg, the uterus will release the lining, which is your monthly period. Then, the whole process starts again.

Endometriosis is a health condition in which the small parts of the lining – the endometrium – begin growing in distinct places, for instance, the ovaries. That can determine the appearance of infertility. The abnormal cell growth may lead to the occurrence of adhesions and cysts. They can barricade your pelvis. This particular aspect will make it almost impossible for the egg to be properly released and afterward facilitate the fertilization process.

This particular condition often causes long, painful periods, irregular bowel movements, and pain during intercourse, and in some cases infertility.

Irregular sperm count and motility

Another quite common cause of infertility is irregular sperm count and motility. If you didn't know it yet, not all sperm can reach and fertilize the egg. It has to be oval-shaped, with a long tail. Irregular sperm has tail or head defects, for instance, a crooked or double tail.

Only the best sperm will reach the egg and fertilize it. Sperm morphology refers to the man's size and shape of the sperm. Typically, this aspect is analyzed to determine a man's fertility. Sperm morphology tests indicate the amount of sperm that is normal when examined under a microscope.

Such a test is done in a laboratory, by a certified specialist. The evaluation of the sperm size, shape, and other specific features is carried out by placing a sperm sample under the microscope. By adding colored "dyes" or stains to the sperm, the observer can differentiate abnormal or normal factors characterizing the sperm. Distinctive forms of human sperm have been distinguished.

They include unusual head, abnormal tail, immature germ cells and, of course, standard forms. The usual one is characterized by an overall head shape, having a single, distinctive tail, and an intact middle. Abnormal heads include a broad range of head irregularities that have been notified; they vary from large – macrocephalic to small – microcephalic, or there are cases in which this part isn't identifiable at all. Broken, double, or triple tails are also recognized as abnormal. The existence of cytoplasmic droplets along the tail may outline the existence of immature sperm.

Your doctor will inform your partner about what he should do in advance of the semen analysis. For best results, one is advised to avoid ejaculation for 24 to 72 hours before taking the test. Taking herbal medicine or hormone medications under the guidance of your medical provider should also be paused. In the case in which the results aren't favorable, your doctor will ask your and your partner to proceed to make a range of additional tests, such as hormone and genetic tests, urinalysis after ejaculation, a tissue sample from the testicles or anti-sperm immune cells testing.

Statistics show us that a lot of men present a considerable high amount of abnormal sperm, which is quite common. And we cannot say that a sperm morphology test clearly shows whether a man is fertile or not. In some cases, the problem of the couple trying to conceive might be a mixture of health conditions, so no general rule applies to every couple. We can say that the quality of the egg is equally significant, but, unfortunately, it cannot be tested. However, specialists say that women who are over 35 are prone to having eggs of poorer quality.

Concerning the number of the sperm, it carries a lot of weight. If you want to stand a chance of fertilizing the egg, during ejaculation, the sperm count has to be above 39 million.

Polycystic Ovarian Syndrome (PCOS)

The woman suffering from polycystic ovarian syndrome is unable to conceive because the entire process of conceiving is prevented due to hormonal imbalance. The small follicles in the ovaries fail to grow into mature follicles that will form the eggs.

The primary symptoms linked to this condition are obesity, acne, irregular periods and abnormal hair growth.

Typically, most women dealing with this condition can conceive after implementing a set of dietary and lifestyle alterations such as a healthy diet and plenty of exercise. Overweight women who aimed at losing weight managed to get pregnant afterward. However, in more severe cases, other medical procedures may be efficient.

Submucosal fibroids

Fibroids are known as non-cancerous tumors that develop in the proximity of the womb or inside of it. In this direction, submucosal fibroids grow inside the womb. In some cases, this condition can diminish the woman's odds of conceiving. It is assumed that the fibroid hinders the embryo from developing inside the womb.

Varicocele

This particular situation might alarm people, but you would be surprised to find out that more than 40 percent of the men coping with infertility suffer from this condition. To be more precise, the man suffering from it presents varicose veins in the scrotum.

In some cases, the condition is not that severe, but in other cases, surgery is required. Another procedure that is growing in popularity, known as embolization, is highly efficient as well and doesn't imply surgery or general anesthesia.

Fallopian tube damage or Blockage

I want to outline the crucial importance of having regular tests for sexually transmitted diseases. While some of these conditions don't even come with stressing symptoms, what most people fail to understand is that they can lead to infertility. For instance, chlamydia and gonorrhea, very ordinary conditions, can contribute to the appearance of the pelvic inflammatory disease.

Pelvic inflammatory disease is a condition that harms your reproductive organs, in this way making it difficult for you to conceive. Sadly, these harmful bacteria affect the fallopian tubes and make it nearly impossible for the sperm to encounter the egg. And, even worse, there are cases in which the egg is fertilized and then gets stuck inside the fallopian tubes. As a result, the uterus grown in size and the fallopian tubes suffer a rupture. This particular condition is known as misplaced carriage – ectopic pregnancy. It's very severe, and it can kill the woman.

Primary ovarian insufficiency

This condition is also referred to as early menopause. The ovaries no longer function as expected, and menstruation ceases to happen before the age of 40. In many cases, the underlying reason for this condition is widely unknown. Nonetheless, it appears that some factors associated with it are radiation, immune system diseases, chemotherapy treatment, and smoking.

Health-related factors and further problems that affect fertility

There are numerous health-related factors that, combined, may lead to hormonal imbalance, low ovarian reserve, poor egg quality, or abnormal immune response to conception. If you recognize that one or more of the following factors feature your lifestyle, you should address these issues as they may have a detrimental influence on your ability to conceive.

- Thyroid issues
- Autoimmune disease
- Poor adrenal health
- Trauma or injury to the reproductive organs
- Alcoholism
- Hypertension
- Long-term medicine intake
- Exposure to pollution and environmental toxins
- Hormonal imbalance linked to infertility

Besides having well-timed sex on a regular basis, your body hormones have to be working in perfect order for you to conceive. Why? Because hormones are the ones that trigger the entire process of conception.

The beginning of a woman's menstrual cycle determines the release of brain signals to the pituitary gland indicating that the body has to release the egg. The luteal phase marks the increase of progesterone levels inside the body. This hormone determines the formation of the uterus' lining for pregnancy. In case the sperm fertilizes the egg, the body continues to produce progesterone. However, when women deal with hormonal imbalances, this process is interrupted.

Ovulation problems are significantly prevalent to the extent that up to 25 percent of women dealing with infertility suffer from this kind of issues. And, in most cases, the triggering root to this problem is a hormonal imbalance.

In most instances, it's your daily life and diet that make your hormones go crazy. Chronic stress, weight loss and gain, even strenuous regular workouts are factors that can mess up your hormonal balance. If something inside your body is not right, then it's only obvious that your hormonal balance is altered as well.

For instance, Polycystic ovarian syndrome (PCOS) is a health condition from which a lot of women suffer. Having this syndrome increases a woman's chances of experiencing a miscarriage with up to 45 percent.

Thyroid disease can be, in some cases, the triggering cause of hormonal imbalances leading to infertility. Thyroid hormones play a major importance for maintaining our overall health. Hyperthyroidism is a health condition that affects the thyroid gland, making it generate more hormones than normal. When fewer hormones than necessary are produced, the condition is known as hypothyroidism. Either condition can seriously harm a woman's hormonal balance, thus lead to infertility. Typically, hypothyroidism is linked with luteal phase dysfunction, determined by an insufficient production of progesterone.

Why does hormonal imbalance occur?

Stress

Among the many things that cause hormonal imbalances, stress is the most obvious and most problematic. At the moment, the modern-paced lifestyle we lead makes us experience plenty of pressure, which imminently leads to sleep disorders and other problems.

There is research pointing that stress increases the levels of hormones, including cortisol in men, which affects the man's release of sex hormones. At the same time, it has an adverse influence on the man's sperm count. Plus, in women, stress prevents ovulation from taking place normally. Chronic stress is also in many cases the source of severe thyroid problems as well as adrenal fatigue. Later on, I will expand on the way in which stress interferes with a couple's ability to conceive.

Bad nutrition

You must perceive your body as if it were a vehicle. Will your car drive you to your wished destination if you don't place the right, high-quality fuel and if you don't get it checked on a regular basis? Certainly not. It might work for a while, but in time, it will be damaged. The same happens with our bodies. They must receive the necessary amounts of vitamins, minerals and nutritive value to function correctly. Would you rely on your car to drive you to work if you don't fuel it up? No. The same way with food; you can't expect to get pregnant and deliver a healthy baby if you don't aim at nurturing your body by eating properly.

Exposure to xenohormones

Xenohormones are chemicals we expose ourselves to on a daily basis. This increased exposure can genuinely interfere with the body's natural ability of conceiving. All these chemicals can be conveyed as endocrine disruptors. Why? Because they can change the way in which the natural hormones are produced. Here comes a list of the most common xenohormones we expose ourselves to:

- Hormonal birth control
- Non-organic meats (the majority of animals are fed with large amounts of hormones to reach maturity faster)
- Plastics
- Pesticides, fungicides, herbicides
- Solvents
- Adhesives
- Emulsifiers present in cosmetics

[29]

- Negative lifestyle choices

Sedentary lifestyles, paired up with high levels of stress and sleep irregularities can also cause hormonal imbalances. When the individuals trying to get pregnant consume increased amounts of sugary foods, alcoholic drinks, smoke or use drugs, conception can be prevented. Also, if a person is taking a particular kind of medication, hormonal release can become abnormal.

Body fat

Body fat cells are known as adipocytes, and they produce estrogen. For this reason, women who don't present an average amount of body fat may encounter hormonal imbalances and infertility. In short, insufficient body fat can trigger ovulation to stop taking place inside the woman's body.

On the other hand, individuals who have higher amounts of body fat present increased amounts of estrogen, which can also lead to infertility. We are talking about estrogen dominance. And this particular aspect applies to both men and women. Men struggling with obesity present lowered testosterone levels. Plus, the sperm of obese men often shows irregularities, which will grow the woman's risks of experiencing miscarriage and chromosol defects. Plus, there are many cases in which overweight men deal with sexual dysfunctions.

Genetics

Ongoing scientific research indicates that there might be a link between infertility problems and genetic predispositions in this direction. For instance, there is a genetic predisposition towards obesity or autoimmune diseases, which in some cases lead to infertility.

Treatment options

Various fertility issues are more easily treated, as opposed to others. Concurrently, factors such as health condition, genetics and age are acknowledged as important as well. Generally speaking, as a woman reaches 35 years old, her likelihood of conceiving slightly decreases.

In this situation, your doctor may recommend you to skip some of the steps young couples are recommended to consider. That's, mainly, because the odds of conceiving diminish with each passing year. Before embracing a particular treatment, it's important to discuss with your partner about the budget, and how far you intend to go – are you opting for medicine, or would you consider insemination or surrogacy, as final alternatives? Fertility treatments can be quite costly, and most of the cases, the insurance doesn't cover these costs.

Fertility treatments – What are your alternatives?

If you're concerned about your apparent inability to conceive, the odds are that a visit to your doctor will provide you with the reassurance and advice you so desperately need. Some couples will require turning to a specialist in assisted conception techniques. In this direction, the following information will give you a brief introduction to the fertility treatments available at the moment so that you can consider your options.

For treating various ovulation problems, one of the treatments available includes clomiphene, which is a drug that stimulates the ovaries to produce the egg for fertilization. Another option is metformin, which is typically administered to women suffering from polycystic ovary syndrome.

For the woman whose fallopian tubes are blocked, an option would be tubal surgery. The operation aims at correcting this common-met health condition, the complication of the intervention depending on the extent of the blockage. After this surgery, you might experience some degree of discomfort in your chest and shoulders, due the carbon dioxide used during the operation. The medical specialist uses carbon dioxide in order to see the organs easily.

In the case in which endometriosis is the primary cause of your infertility, a readily available treatment is laparoscopic surgery, whose purpose is to remove the endometrial tissue growth. Nonetheless, this treatment cannot be considered as a viable alternative if your condition is severe.

Fertility drugs such as clomifene pills and gonadotrophin injections aim at regulating the production of hormones, as well as triggering the release of an egg per cycle. The success rate? Nearly 29 percent birth rate acknowledged for clomifene, and 20 percent for gonadotrophin injections. Side effects for clomifene include mood swings, hot flushes, vaginal dryness and breast tenderness. On the other hand, gonadotrophin injections lead to headaches, soreness, digestive issues or bloating.

Intrauterine insemination – your partner's or a donor's sperm is injected into your uterus through a flexible tube or a catheter. Afterward, the sperm sample will be pretreated, in order to extract the best quality sperm. The success rate of this procedure is 15 percent.

In vitro fertilization is another frequently-met procedure nowadays. As infertility rates are on the growth, more and more couples consider this alternative. Let me explain how it works. First, a doctor will remove the eggs from your ovaries. Next, the eggs will be fertilized in a laboratory, and afterward, the doctor will allow them to grow into embryos. The next step is transferring the eggs back in the uterus. The success rate of this procedure is 32 percent. What else should you know? Fertility drugs you might be administered as part of the treatment may lead to an array of unpleasant side effects.

Intracytoplasmic sperm injection – a single sperm will be injected into a particular egg. The embryo that will result afterward will be transferred into the uterus. This medical procedure is similar to in vitro fertilization. The doctor may require collecting a sperm sample from your partner's testicle, by making a tiny cut, or an injection.

[32]

Donor insemination – donor sperm is typically used for fertilizing an egg via intrauterine insemination. You might feel discouraged, and experience a sense of inadequacy, by not having a baby who shares both your genes and your partner's.

Egg or embryo donation – another woman donates an egg, and, after being fertilized, it is transferred into your uterus.

Surrogacy – another woman will carry the baby for you. After his/her birth, you and your partner are legally recognized as parents. The fetus may result from an embryo made from your egg and your partner's sperm, or from a donor. You may not feel at ease with this alternative because you cannot control what the mother eats, and how she handles stress. These are factors that have a significant impact on the baby's development. By all means, it's recommended to pick a person you can communicate with easily, and that you can trust 100 percent.

What are the odds of conceiving with fertility treatments?

A significant number of women who encounter difficulties in conceiving are prescribed clomiphene citrate – which is an oral drug provoking ovulation. Nearly 35 percent of the women who were administered this medication became pregnant in the course of a treatment of six cycles. In the cases in which fertility drugs are combined with IUI, for instance, pregnancy rates naturally grow. However, the success rate imminently depends on the seriousness of the problem, your health history, genetics, and age.

What about the success rates you keep hearing about? Are they truly reliable? Before considering any treatment, it is important to factor in the success rates. But think of them as having an informative purpose, as these numbers are based on national averages. For instance, your doctor may recommend a different treatment after a certain amount of time, because each couple's problem is different, and should be treated individually, as such. As always, I will repeat myself by saying that you shouldn't compare your case with any others.

Which is the latest controversial study regarding infertility?

As scientists are eagerly working towards acquiring valuable information regarding effective treatments for infertility, a team of researchers from Spain has managed to create human sperm successfully, from skin cells. That is acknowledged as a medical feat that may eventually lead to establishing a new treatment for infertility. Nonetheless, the issue is quite controversial.

The aim was to find an efficient solution for those couples who couldn't conceive, and whose sole alternative was donated sperm and eggs. Hence, they addressed the root of the problem, by creating gametes in the people that don't have them. The research was developed at Stanford University, in the United States, and was afterward published in Scientific Reports, the online journal of *Nature*.

The team of researchers succeeded to reprogram mature skin cells, as they introduced the cells required to create the gametes. In a month's time, the skin cell developed into a germ cell, which can further develop into either an egg or sperm. Nonetheless, according to their findings, it didn't have the capability to fertilize.

Carlos Simon, the leading researcher, noted that the result was a sperm that needs an additional maturation phase, in an attempt to turn into a gamete, affirming that this is the initial stage of a fruitful research. The researchers must consider legal constraints as well, as the technique implies creating artificial embryos, which, at the time being, is permitted only in some countries. Hence, we're talking about a lengthy process.

Chapter 3: Fertility – How It's Perceived in Different Cultures and What is Its Link with the Educational System

In this chapter, you will learn:

- How different cultures perceive fertility
- The link between sex education and fertility
- What are the main differences concerning fertility in different cultures?

Fertility is a subject that is highly influenced by a range of external factors – cultural, religious and socioeconomic. An important question is the following – do cultural variables genuinely affect this sector of our lives, and if yes, to what extent?

In order to comprehend human fertility rates and the discrepancies that imminently emerge, one should aim at outlining cultural influences. A range of questions might arise – how come that, in spite of advanced means of communication, and the amount of information readily available, there are still cultures with large families of children, even though they confront with starvation? Why, in some cultures, governmental birth control efforts haven't come down to a fruitful result?

For instance, in the Islamic cultures, a range of strict pro-fertility patterns lie at the foundation of the society. Children are desired because large families in these cultures are highly-appraised, as opposed to others. There are various cultural and religious meanings that childbearing carries in Islamic cultures. Nonetheless, it appears that contraception is legal, in some countries such as Pakistan and Egypt. Surprisingly, though, in Turkey, this concept wasn't acclaimed. The distinct practices within these cultures are explained through political motives, as opposed to religious ones, as you might be inclined to assume. There are also some paradoxical situations. An example is that of Turkey, which hasn't legalized contraception. However, it is resistant towards penalizing abortionists. In the same respects, Israel has legalized contraception, but harshly punishes abortions.

Unquestionably, lack of information and communication between spouses concerning childbirth and sex are the main characteristics in the vast majority of sociocultural groups in underdeveloped countries. Even if literacy and education are existing factors, accurate information concerning reproduction is shrouded in ignorance, or, even worse, the information concerning birth control isn't reliable because it's derived from untrusted sources.

Such cultural premises refer to puritanical approaches by husbands and wives who are ashamed to discuss these matters. There's the modesty concept, in some cultures, according to which women won't consider a physical examination by a male physician, some being ashamed to be contemplated by their own husbands. Such examples are vivid in areas in which population growth rates are high, in Islamic countries, India, and Latin America.

Concerning African birth rates, they are typically high, as children symbolize old age security and prestige. The practice of polygamy also enables an individual to father a significant number of children. There are cases in which, perhaps, both the husband and wife have knowledge of contraceptive methods, but, as their cultural and religious beliefs hamper their freedom, they won't consider these alternatives as viable.

Certainly, another crucial factor of importance is education. Education is primordial for disseminating reliable birth control methods to control population increases. However, in some regions, education is sometimes blocked by cultural customs and values.

[36]

It's acknowledged that in the cases in which women have access to education, and paid employment opportunities, pregnancy rates are significantly lower. As mentioned above, career prospects put a hold on family planning. However, in developing countries, women that don't pursue education will have two or more children than women with secondary school education. Additionally, families in developing countries rely on having numerous children that would support them at old age, as opposed to civilized countries where individuals benefit from private and public pension systems. In rural areas, children are conveyed as a crucial part of the labor force, aiding their parents from a very early age.

We observe a range of striking discrepancies. The Western World copes with infertility issues, as the educational focus has been, almost entirely, directed towards contraceptive methods. On the other hand, in underdeveloped countries, due to a mixture of cultural and religious motives, the reality differs, resulting in overpopulation matters in an environment in which starvation is a frequently-met issue.

Sex education and fertility – is there a missing link in the educational system?

It would appear that, at the moment, when it comes to sex education, the primary focus is directed towards teaching teenagers what they should do in order to avoid pregnancy and sexually transmitted diseases, at all costs. As a result, whether it's done willingly or not, the stressing issue of fertility is left out entirely, which leaves the greater majority of the population uninformed and unaware of its limitations.

Clinics are filled with women who, given a wide range of reasons, couldn't conceive naturally. Whether we're talking about couples who found one another a bit late or women with rollercoaster careers that didn't permit them to focus on something else, the reality is striking. That leads us to one question - what is a common factor these women in clinics share? Awareness of their fertility limitations.

Many women who arrive in this position, acknowledging that the clock is ticking, and the likelihood of conceiving diminishes with each passing day, affirm that they wish they have known that age is such a triggering factor for fertility. And, contrary to what you may assume, I'm not talking about uneducated women – I'm referring to smart, confident women, who have built amazing careers. But, unfortunately, they lacked a solid education concerning fertility.

Currently, sex education in school is delivered – and that is a positive aspect – to keep teenagers informed, and maintain teenage pregnancy rates low. Nonetheless, the problem is that emphasis is placed, almost entirely, on avoiding pregnancy and catching sexually-transmitted diseases. As a result, the incidence of teenage pregnancies has diminished, but, at the same time, the striking reality is that one in six couples deals with infertility. What's the link between these two instances? By aiming at encouraging teenagers to avoid pregnancy, they seem to miss that, with age, fertility diminishes, slightly, yet steadily.

Consequently, many women end up in a private clinic, being struck by the cruel irony of having spent years avoiding pregnancy, and when they're ready to make that step, things don't seem to work out as they expect them to. The truth is that something's missing – fertility education.

The primary distinction between sexual health education and fertility introduction is that the former is directed towards the present while the second is meant for the future. Something young women should comprehend is that, with time, the number of eggs decreases. I have notice that many women had come across this information only later on, when they considered pregnancy, and it was already a bit late. Luckily, they did manage to conceive, but with numerous sacrifices.

Concurrently, boys and girls need to acknowledge that a broad range of external factors has a significant impact on fertility as well, such as smoking, alcohol, drugs and sexually transmitted diseases.

The bottom-line? This generation needs to be given an adequate education concerning fertility, in order to comprehend that pregnancy depends on many factors, and it doesn't always happen when one expects. Hence, there's a missing link in our reproductive educational system. It's important to deliver a balanced mindset, so that young people comprehend that pregnancy is a complex phenomenon, and treat it as such.

Chapter 4: Reverse Infertility by Making Lifestyle and Dietary Changes

In this chapter, you will learn:

- How to reverse infertility by changing your eating habits.
- What lifestyle changes you should make.

If you wish to increase your odds of getting pregnant and cure infertility, there are certain changes you should consider making. Most of the times, the reason a woman might not be getting pregnant is not necessarily infertility. As a matter of fact, in the greater majority of infertility cases, the body can genuinely reverse infertility if you give it the appropriate resources.

I have worked with plenty of women who were going through emotional struggle because they thought they were unable to conceive and fought will all kinds of negative feelings and emotions. Still, the good news for you is that, the majority of women I've worked with managed to get pregnant after considering some lifestyle changes. There's no sacrifice too big for having your baby, is there?

Lifestyle changes, while they might be quite difficult to implement, at first, are useful, and from my personal experience, they work 100 percent of the time. It is needless to say that they cost significantly less than other infertility cures.

Infertility is quite a complex issue, which sometimes has quite simple solutions. There is a myriad of factors that range from every couple in particular and, combined, can lead to infertility. Therefore, conventional treatments are rarely effective, plus they may have a variety of side effects. My experience in the domain has shown me that every woman who deeply yearns to hold her baby in her arms can make that a reality if she puts her mind to changing her lifestyle.

What determines infertility?

There is no general definition of infertility that applies to every woman or couple. It can be caused by a myriad of factors including hormonal imbalance, physical blockage, shortage of luteinizing hormone, inadequate hormonal production, and many other factors. As I said, this problem is quite complex and differs from every woman or couple. I have already mentioned the most commonly met health problems linked to infertility.

However, what seems to apply to the greater majority of couples is that poor nutrition combined with increased exposure to harmful toxins can also cause infertility. Take a moment to consider your lifestyle, your eating habits, whether you engage in sporting activities or not, and other factors as well. Believe it or not, the way in which you live your life can determine whether you'll be expecting a baby soon or not. Thus, making lifestyle and dietary changes can genuinely help you increase your fertility and, at the same time, will help you live a healthier and happier life.

Reverse Infertility

Nutrition

For starters, this is probably the most important aspect you should take into consideration. Besides the common problem of getting overweight, this is also one of the triggering factors that lead to infertility, our modern dietary habits lead to undernourished bodies. Take it like this; your body is genuinely unable to permit the development of a pregnancy if it's unprepared for it, as it doesn't have the necessary foundation. Your body cannot nurture a pregnancy if it's typically unable to care for itself, to put it roughly.

[41]

Diet is genuinely the most important factor that will aid you to support fertility health. What you eat plays a majestic role in the formation of the cells that make the eggs and the sperm. You are what you eat. What do you usually eat? If you usually eat processed foods and lots of sugary meals, then you've found the root of your problem. A nutritional deficiency can be the primary triggering factor that causes an irregular menstrual cycle. If you find you have trouble monitoring what you eat on a regular basis, I recommend you try keeping a journal in which you write everything you eat during a day. This way, you will know exactly what you put inside your body and where you need to make adjustments.

A lot of women deal with weight problems, and, as a result might turn to weight-loss programs, which might be valid to some extent, but still won't solve the real issue. While there are studies that indicate that weight loss contributes to increasing fertility, your body needs to be properly taken care of and carefully nourished as well. On the other hand, if you're too thin, or you're dealing or have dealt in the past with anorexia or bulimia, getting a healthful, nutritious diet plays such a crucial role. What you need to understand is that for a healthy hormone production, your body needs its set of healthy proteins and fats.

This is why I've come up with the following list concerning nutrition so that you understand what dietary changes you need to make. It might be difficult, at first, to change your dietary habits, but, trust me, it's a necessity, and it will bring you so much closer to becoming the proud mother of a beautiful baby. Next, I would like to present to you the all-natural fertility diet you should follow for maximizing your fertility.

#1 Eliminate processed foods

Consider eliminating processed foods, artificial sugary items and starches from your daily diet. Your body requires carbohydrates, but it needs to get them from healthy sources such as vegetables, fruits and sweet potatoes and squash, which are positive additions to your diet.

#2 Include more healthy fats into your diet

Add more healthy fats in your diet from sources such as coconut oil, olives and olive oil, butter, eggs, avocado, and nuts.

#3 Eat more protein

Make sure you eat plenty of protein to ensure your body's health. Use sources such as eggs, nuts, and grass-fed meats. Organic, grass-fed meat may appear like a novelty to you. That's why I want to clarify the reasons I recommend it.

You should choose grass-fed meat over conventional meat due to numerous reasons. For starters, various studies prove us that grass-fed meat is richer in nutrients, having a significant impact on boosting fertility as well. Studies of nearly three decades indicate that grass-fed meat is filled with essential fatty acids, containing a diverse range of powerful antioxidants, and has a lower intake of fat, compared to other types of meat.

In fact, it does make sense that these animals are healthy, as they aren't exposed to numerous detrimental factors that may harm the quality of their meat. Of course, we shouldn't miss including the ethical reason as well – these animals are raised in positive environments, as opposed to others, living in cramped settings, and being fed God-knows-what. Hence, when you have the possibility to choose, make sure to make the right decision for the sake of your health, and your future baby.

#4 Avoid processed foods

Avoid anti-nutritive foods, more precisely, processed foods. Our diets, sadly, abound with these artificial, quick meals that are easy to prepare. But please try and replace them. The chemicals found in these meals can consequently disrupt your hormonal balance.

#5 Avoid processed dairy items

Steer clear of eating processed dairy items. Instead, opt for raw, organic dairy product such as butter and heavy cream which don't contain additional chemicals.

#6 Regular insulin levels

Having your insulin levels under control is crucial as well. Insulin resistance often accompanies a diet rich in carbohydrates. Optimizing your diet by taking into account the enumerated methods will grow your body's sensitivity to insulin, thus increase your hormone production and lead to the proper functioning of your body.

#7 Eat more fruits and vegetables

Fruits and vegetables – you should consider having, at least, five to eight servings of fruits and veggies a day. Eat as many fruits and vegetables as needed. You can choose to eat them either raw or steamed, to preserve their right functions. My personal advice is to mix the colors of the fruits and veggies you have so that you combine a range of vitamins and nutrients.

Did you know that the color of the fruit or vegetable can indicate its nutritional content? For instance, orange and yellow fruit servings are loaded with beta-carotene. So, don't hesitate to include delicious fruits including apricots, peaches, nectarines, papaya, cantaloupe, carrots.

Vitamin C is also extremely important, being a potent antioxidant. Apples and citrus fruits are filled with the necessary amounts of vitamin C. Thus, having a freshly-squeezed orange juice in the morning, is definitely a positive idea! Other fruits rich in antioxidant compounds are berries and the best part about them is that they contain little amounts of sugar. Add to your diet blackberries, raspberries, strawberries, cranberries, blueberries, and boysenberries. Of course, you shouldn't overlook green leafy veggies that are filled with valuable minerals your body requires. Opt for spinach, kale, radicchio, lettuce, and other greenery veggies.

#8 Cut back on desserts and refined sugars

Cut back on sweets and refined sugars. If you have a sweet tooth, I feel sorry to tell you that you need to eliminate any sugary servings from your diet, as excess sugar in the bloodstream can contribute to preventing the body from manufacturing the reproduction hormones. My personal recommendation to you is to try to replace these for the sake of your health. Opt for fruits instead of desserts and plan a day of the week when you spoil yourself with a yummy cake, but nothing more than that. I bake a lot of muffins or pies with organic ingredients and more fruits, you can also try that. Don't be resistant to trying new recipes.

For some women, optimizing nutrition is all it takes to get pregnant. Still, even if you do succeed to get pregnant after you include these dietary changes in your life, don't give in by returning to your old habits. A proper nutrition plays a crucial role in delivering a healthy baby and preventing miscarriage. According to my vast experience in this field, one of the triggering factors that lead to infertility is a diet lacking in healthy fats and proteins. Your body is practically unable to produce hormones if it's not given a proper diet.

Lifestyle changes

It's no secret that negative habits such as lack of sleep, smoking or high caffeine intake can be triggering factors that prevent women from conceiving. Every doctor will confirm that these aspects can be the reasons for your infertility.

#1 Get enough sleep

Don't underestimate the importance of having a regular sleeping schedule. If you didn't know it before, sleep plays a significant role in the production of hormones. According to

[45]

studies developed in this domain, women who had low melatonin and serotonin levels presented a shorter luteal phase. The luteal phase is, typically, the amount of time between ovulation and menstruation. Therefore, if the luteal phase is shortened, your chances of becoming pregnant are significantly diminished. Additionally, sleep deprivation also reduces the body's capability to regulate adrenaline, insulin, and cortisone. This particular aspect will make conception hard to achieve.

I recommend you consider sleep a priority and make sure you feel perfectly well-rested after you wake up in the morning. Sometimes, this might mean taking a nap during the day. Another tip of advice if you're dealing with insomnia would be to make sure your room is dark during the night. You can get some dark-colored curtains, for instance. That might come in quite handy.

#2 Limit exposures to harmful toxins

Try not to expose yourself to harmful toxins. The majority of women I've talked to indicated significant improvements once they've slowly eliminated household chemicals, conventional cosmetics, and plastic containers and so on and so forth.

#3 Exercise

As cliché as it may sound, the proper amount of exercise is the key to a healthy lifestyle. And a healthy lifestyle is the solution to getting pregnant. You see where I'm headed, don't you? Consider introducing exercise into your daily routine. Consider taking up fun sports that you enjoy such as tennis, swimming, or other weight-loss programs. You need to engage yourself in any movement, long strolls in the forest, for instance, or walking your dog around the neighborhood. If you're also dealing with insomnia, exercise can help you solve that issue as well, as it improves circulation, decreases blood pressure and gets you in a good mood.

However, do make sure not to force it, when I'm saying that exercising will improve your chances of getting pregnant, I'm not referring to training for a running marathon, if you know what I mean! Studies show us that women who engaged in vigorous forms of exercise had significantly lower chances of getting pregnant.

#4 If you are under medication, talk to a doctor

Additionally, you should consider talking to your doctor if you're taking medications, say for a particular medical condition you may have. This way, he/she can determine whether that could deter you from conceiving. You should know that taking steroids and antidepressants can detrimentally affect the hormone productions in your body, thus leading to infertility.

#5 Quit smoking

Smoking can harmfully affect fertility in both men and women. The harmful chemicals that are found in cigarettes including nicotine, carbon monoxide and genuinely contribute to the loss rate of a woman's eggs, and a man's fertility as well. The man plays quite an important role in the equation! Thus, please stay away from smoking of any sort, recreational smoking as well.

#6 Quit drinking coffee in excess

Studies show that women who intake large amounts of caffeine on a regular basis are less likely to become pregnant compared to other women. Thus, consider reducing the amount of caffeine you drink. Normally, according to research, one cup of coffee a day is not harmful. Try not to exceed that.

#7 Give up alcohol

It is recommendable for women who wish to get pregnant to give up alcohol. It can genuinely lower your odds of conceiving, even if you don't drink heavily massive amounts of tequila. Also, once you've managed to get pregnant, make sure not to sip alcoholic beverages, but most probably you already know that.

Supplements

From my experience, including the dietary and lifestyle changes above can make a world of a difference if you're trying to have a baby. Still, other methods could help you to achieve your purpose if those changes alone won't live up to the task. Some women have told me that after taking some natural herbal supplements, they enjoyed faster results. In this view, it's imperative to take omega-3 supplements that will provide your body with the nutrients and fatty acids it requires.

I used to take them during pregnancy and before, during the nursing period as well, to make sure that the baby is getting all the necessary nutrients. There are other herbal supplements I used to take as well, and I will enumerate them below. However, there are supplements that plenty of women have taken and affirmed that they're extremely helpful.

#1 Nettle Leaf

It is rich in minerals while being filled with chlorophyll that is genuinely nourishing to the kidneys in particular. As a matter of fact, Nettle Leaf contributes to reducing stress, while being an effective uterine tonic. During pregnancy, it is genuinely helpful as well, as it is filled with extraordinary amounts of vitamin K, which will help to prevent bleeding. It tastes great, and it can cure infertility both in men and women. This tea will also boost your levels of calcium, vitamin A, and C. I add nettle leaf to tea, and my advice is to drink it before and during pregnancy.

#2 Red raspberry leaf tea

It is probably the most favorite tea when it comes to curing infertility. Similar to nettle leaf, it is also an ideal source of essential minerals and vitamins – A, B-complex, C, E and significant levels of phosphorus and potassium. I recommend it to couples who have been trying to get pregnant for a while now, as this tea is mainly known for its effectiveness. It tones the uterus while being famous among herbalists for reducing the pain of the contractions during labor.

#3 Dandelion

Dandelion is recommended especially for its amazing detoxifying properties. It can contribute to aiding your body in eliminating harmful toxins. Additionally, it contains vitamins A and C and supports the health of the liver.

#4 Maca

Maca is a herb that presents the function of balancing the hormonal production in the body, being widely popular for its effectiveness. It can be taken both by men and women. Maca promotes the proper functioning of the reproductive system, supporting the hormonal balance, which is, usually, the triggering factor of infertility.

Rumor has it that ancient local people living around the area known today as Peru settled that a single plant increased the fertility to their herds. This plant is known as maca root, which, in some cases is eaten as a vegetable, being similar to broccoli and cabbage. As a result, locals began eating this plant for this purpose, and not only, because it is also known to improve memory function and energy. This was common especially in the Andes region, where this plant grows extensively. At the moment, maca root referred to as Peruvian ginseng, is acknowledged all over the world for its fertility boosting capabilities.

To begin with, maca root is believed to be an aphrodisiac. Typically, it should grow the frequency of sexual intercourse, having a great impact on fertility. While it is true that this root includes some compounds that may have a positive influence in this direction, these assumptions are not entirely accurate and not all of them have been researched thoroughly. However, being a natural ingredient, you can safely use maca as a fertility boost.

The all-natural fertility diet – what should you be eating for optimal fertility?

Having a fertility diet for preparing your body for pregnancy is primordial, and possibly, the first thing you can do for your baby. Multiple studies indicate us that particular lifestyle and dietary changes can function as fertility boost and prevent miscarriage and birth defects. Think of the process of getting pregnant as if you were preparing for a most awaited vacation. You have to prepare a lot for everything to go well, right? The same principle applies here. An all-natural fertility diet should be the first thing on your mind if you wish to conceive!

Every time I asked a couple about their dietary choices, their responses were positively saying "they're healthy." Nonetheless, as they further expanded on their notion of healthy, I realized that what appears to be healthy to some may not be such a fertility-friendly diet. Because a fertility diet differs from a healthy one.

When I'm talking about a fertility diet, I'm referring to a diet that supports the correct functioning of the reproductive system. It consists of foods that are rich in particular nutrients and can ensure the proper hormonal production, fetal development, sperm and egg health, blood health and so on. This diet will help the body dealing with infertility issues surpass them while ensuring the health of the baby to be born. This diet is your way of making sure that your baby will enter this world healthy and joyful.

Why should you opt for a fertility diet?

- Deficiencies in particular nutrients can trigger the appearance of birth defects.
- The foods you and your partner eat have a significant impact on the health of the sperm and egg.
- Hormonal imbalance is, in most cases, caused by a bad diet.
- The triggering cause to anovulation is an improper diet.

[50]

Harvard University developed a research that indicated specific improvements in couples who implemented a fertility diet in their lives. Women who included some lifestyle changes, along with altering their diet, presented 80 percent fewer infertility risks. The women who had the highest fertility scores were the ones who ate moderate amounts of trans fats and sugars, consumed more veggies than animal meat, took multivitamins and supplements and opted for high-fat dairy products.

Mother Nature offers us everything our bodies need to keep them nourished and healthy. When we are taking proper care of our body and provide it with everything it needs, it will be able to repair itself.

The primary benefits associated with a fertility diet

- Provides the body with the needed antioxidants, minerals, and vitamins that ensure the health of the egg and sperm.
- Provides the body's hormonal balance by providing the right fat intake.
- Can contribute to diminishing the chances of experiencing miscarriage and giving birth to an ill child.
- Helps constructing the needed nutritive support for each particular pregnancy stage.
- It promotes the correct functioning of the reproductive system.
- It's within everybody's reach.

Fertility diet guidelines

#1 Opt for organic fruits and vegetables

Typically, the greater majority of vegetables and fruits are filled with herbicides and pesticides. In this direction, both female and male fertility is detrimentally affected by the consumption of such foods. For this reason, consider organic fruits and veggies that are 100 percent natural and provide the body with all the vitamins and minerals it requires.

[51]

#2 Have organic, whole fat dairy products

When talking about milk products, opting for full fat, organic products are your best pick. For some women, dairy products can present a negative influence in cases of PCOS and Endometriosis, harming the body's hormonal balance. Thus, it is important that you pay attention to the way in which your body reacts to such foods. Fat-free dairy that is also non-organic is filled with additional hormones and sugar, which will affect the body's hormonal levels. You can consider opting for almond milk instead if that seems more appealing to you.

#3 Opt for grass-fed and organic meat

Generally speaking, you should know that meat coming from conventionally raised animals includes antibiotics and hormones. This can seriously interfere with the body's hormonal secretion. On the other side, though, grass-fed meat encompasses specific beneficial fatty acids, which are a significant protein source. Ideally, you should purchase meat from local farms.

#4 Opt for whole grains, in their natural form

Unprocessed whole grains encompass a great deal of significant vitamins, fiber, and nutrients that support the body's immunity. Whole grain intake is required for a proper digestive function as well as for maintaining the blood sugar balance in order. On the other hand, steer clear of refined white foods and grains, including white bread, white rice, and semolina pasta. Opt for brown rice, whole wheat bread, and whole wheat pasta instead.

#5 Eat more foods rich in fiber

Foods rich in fiber control healthy blood sugar levels which will contribute to diminishing fertility problems, including immunological problems and PCOS. Some excellent alternatives to foods rich in fiber are beans, fruits and vegetables.

#6 Opt for cold water fish

Implementing plenty of fish in your diet is essential as it is an ideal source of omega three fatty acids. They play a crucial role in hormone production, diminishing inflammation, and ensuring a regular menstrual cycle. Fish encompasses critical levels of protein and vitamin A. However, given the fact that some large deep water fish are prone to containing large amounts of mercury, avoid them, and stick to cold water fish. Also, another tip would be opting for wild salmon over farmed salmon because the second one encompasses antibiotics and toxic food dye.

#7 Drink more fresh water

My piece of advice would be to steer clear of bottled water. Why? Because the plastics in the bottle can lead to specific hormonal imbalances due to the harmful chemicals. For this reason, consider clean, purified water, and don't forget to drink at least 2 liters a day. Hydration is crucial for supporting the body's health and oxygenating the brain, so don't overlook it.

Essential foods for boosting fertility

#1 Eggs

Always opt for fresh, organic eggs. While they may cost you a little bit more, they are worth the extra money as they offer you plenty of protein and vitamin intake. The best place from where you should purchase them is the farmer's market or local farms.

#2 Nuts and seeds

Various types of nuts are essential for your health as they are filled with omega 3 fatty acids, vitamin E, Zinc, and protein. But remember to eat them in their raw form to preserve their nutritional value. Walnuts, chia seeds, flax seeds and hemp seeds are excellent sources of omega 3 fatty acids. On the other hand, pumpkin seeds and sesame are highly recommended for their significant zinc and iron intake. Vitamin E is present in almonds and sunflower seeds.

#3 Colorful veggies

As silly as it may sound, the color of the vegetables you eat, in most cases, will show the nutrients and vitamins they contain. For instance, red and green colored veggies are filled with vitamin C, while orange colored ones contain extraordinary levels of vitamin A. To have a balanced diet and make sure that your body receives everything it needs, include a great variety of veggies in your meals. An excellent way to achieve this is to prepare a smoothie in which you add plenty of vegetables and fruits. It tastes great, and it's crazy healthy!

#4 Grass-fed meats

As I already mentioned, you should avoid at all cost buying meat coming from conventionally raised animals. Instead, grass-fed meats are an excellent option because they contain protein, iron, vitamin B12 and omega 3. These animals have been raised without additional antibiotics and harmful hormones that may modify their meat.

#5 Fruits

Typically, fruits contain the largest composition of antioxidants. I suggest you add more prunes, raisins, strawberries, pomegranates, and blueberries to your diet as they are filled with potent natural antioxidants. And remember always to eat your fruit servings fresh.

#6 Liver

If you're not a big fan of liver, you might not be pleased that I added it to this list. But, don't underestimate the amazing impact liver can have on your health. This ingredient is rich in vitamin D, folic acid, B12, iron and zinc. You should try cooking it in various ways until you find that perfect method that suits your taste. It's worth the effort.

#7 Raw dairy

Typically, raw milk products are those products that have not gone through the whole process of pasteurization. That means that they have managed to retain their high amount of enzymes and nutrients. Plus, these foods come from grass-fed cows that weren't fed antibiotics. It's 100 percent safe and even recommended for mothers to be to include raw milk into their diet. You shouldn't do this if you are allergic to it, of course.

#8 Lentils and beans

Lentils and other beans are ideal for the incredible nutritional value they have. If you didn't know it yet, lentils are the second highest food in iron out there and are also an excellent source of folic acid. So, stimulate your cooking creativity and make sure to have plenty of lentils and beans in your meals. You can make cream soups, hummus, or anything you may find appealing.

#9 Fish

Eating fish is possibly one of the greatest favors you can do to your body. It is rich in fatty acids, vitamin D, B12, zinc, CoQ10 and selenium. However, you should bear in mind that this abundance of nutrients is heat-sensitive. Plus, always pay attention to the source of the fish, and opt for those coming from cold water.

#10 Dark, leafy vegetables

Dark, leafy vegetables shouldn't miss from your diet as well. They consist of antioxidants, minerals, and vitamins that support your body's health and wellbeing. Such veggies include kale, spinach, Swiss chard and collards.

Foods to avoid

Soy foods

Soy foods have been recently proven to present a negative impact on a couple's chances of conceiving. For this reason, try to avoid foods including soy milk, soy chips, soy meat, soy burger, soy protein powder and so on and so forth. Research shows us that both men and women are negatively affected by soy products. But what makes soy products so detrimental? The consumption of soy foods actually interferes with the body's natural functioning because they are genetically modified. In the U.S, about 54 percent of the soybeans cultivated in 2005 were acknowledged to be genetically modified. Five years later, 93 percent of the soybeans were genetically modified. You get the picture.

Processed soy foods present significant amounts of aluminum that has a negative effect on the couple's fertility. It appears that soy foods encompass a particular kind of phytoestrogen which is also referred to as isoflavones. Isoflavones present in soy are genistein and daidzein. Some behave similarly to weak estrogen while others as an antiestrogen, which means that they diminish the hormonal production. In this direction, scientists have uncovered that this compound found in soy can decrease fertility. While it is true that there is still research that should be conducted in this area for establishing the truth, the bottom line is that you should be avoiding soy products if you have encountered difficulties in conceiving.

Genetically-modified foods

Research points us that genetically-modified foods can become a stressing problem especially for couples who are yearning to become parents. It appears that this particular issue causes infertility problems at a global rate. Since the 1970s, sperm quality seems to have drastically diminished, and it is estimated that GMO foods are one of the triggering factors of the problem. In spite of the knowledge concerning this subject, manufacturers still use GMOs in producing foods. Now, let's see what makes these foods so harmful for a couple trying to conceive.

Studies developed in the animals' reaction to GMO foods were alarming. A report indicates that the testicles of some animals had a different color after consuming those foods. Plus, the effectiveness of male sperm significantly reduced, resulting in fewer pregnancies. Not to mention that DNA modifications were noticed after the introduction of these foods.

However, males were not the only ones who suffered from the side effects of GMO foods. Female animals encountered infertility problems while the risks associated with premature births increased.

Fat-free foods

You might assume that sticking to fat-free products will help you keep your weight under control. Wrong! As a matter of fact, what often remains under the covers is that, in order to decrease the amount of fat these products contain, they go through a lot of processing and, instead, are filled with sugar. For this reason, avoid fat-free foods, and opt for natural foods that contain normal levels of fat. Fat consumed in reasonable amounts is recommended, for supporting a proper hormonal production.

Sodas and pasteurized juices

Sodas contain high levels of sugar, and they're anything but natural. On the contrary, they can genuinely harm your health. The same goes with pasteurized juices. While you may assume that they should contain 100 percent fruit, that's hardly true in most cases. The greater majority of bottled juices encompass concentrated sugar, which will have a negative impact on your blood sugar levels, immunity, and overall health condition. Sugar itself can be quite harmful as well, so, try replacing it with some natural alternatives such as organic honey, stevia, and maple syrup.

Dangerous fats

While it is true that including plenty of fats in your diet is essential for ensuring your overall health and hormonal balance, unhealthy fats should be avoided at all costs. I'm referring to the fats that lie in delicious, tempting snacks such as donuts, chocolate, chips fries, candy, pies and other similar addictive foods that genuinely affect your health and fertility.

Scientists honestly suggest women wishing to get pregnant to steer clear of all these fats. Make sure you always check the label of every product before purchasing it. Fats you should avoid at all costs are known as "hydrogenated fat," "hardened vegetable fat."

Vitamins promoting fertility

#1 Folic Acid

As I already mentioned, folic acid is required for pregnancy to prepare the body for nurturing the baby and preventing possible complications. For instance, this vitamin is known to prevent congenital heart defects and urinary tract abnormalities from occurring. Plus, folic acid deficiency may grow the risks of preterm birth and other issues such as fetal growth retardation. In some cases, this gap has contributed to spontaneous abortions and pregnancy complications. For this reason, it is best to take it for a couple of months before getting pregnant, and during pregnancy as well. Folic acid promotes ovulation and cell division. For women who are looking to get pregnant, doctors recommend taking 2.000 milligrams a day.

#2 Vitamin D

Vitamin D insufficiency is not uncommon nowadays, particularly during the cold season. The bad news is that vitamin D deficiency presents detrimental effects on the body's health. According to research, there might be a link between infertility and insufficient vitamin D intake. I recommend you consider having a check-up so that you know what health condition you have.

#3 Zinc

Zinc is quite helpful in cell division, sperm production, and ovulation as well. Inside the woman's body, an average of 300 enzymes is regulated by zinc for maintaining the body healthily. Without the necessary zinc intake, the cells are unable to divide. Plus, insufficient zinc is known to lead to miscarriage in the first trimester of pregnancy. However, zinc is necessary for men as well. Infertile men who were given zinc supplements experienced better sperm quality and motility, in this way, increasing their fertility. Given its crucial importance, consider taking zinc supplements accompanied by B-complex vitamins.

#4 B Vitamins

B vitamins insufficiency is quite common especially in people with unhealthy dietary habits, filled with sugar, processed foods, and grains. I recommend you consider B vitamins supplements because they are proven to grow the levels of luteinizing hormone, thus contributing to preventing infertility.

#5 Vitamin C

Active vitamin C levels contribute to enhancing hormone levels and fertility as well, especially in women suffering from luteal phase defect. Vitamin C is a wonderful antioxidant that is recommended for infertility both in men and women. For men, vitamin C contributes to the improvement of the sperm and its motility, while preventing DNA damage from occurring. The recommended dosage is 2.000 milligrams.

#6 Selenium

Selenium is an essential compound that strengthens the body against the harmful effects of free radicals and oxidative stress. It also contributes to guarding the egg and sperm, being famous for helping with cell division. Studies developed in infertile men showed that they had low levels of selenium.

Top health tips that grow male fertility

Typically, when a couple experiences fertility issues, the primary focus is put on the woman. Not so fast. Studies show us that men can also be the source of the problem when conception doesn't happen.

It is only obvious that the man plays a crucial role in conception, right? You don't have to be a rocket scientist to find that out. It is essential that the man's sperm lives long enough inside the woman's body so that it fertilizes the egg waiting inside the fallopian tubes. For the egg to be fertilized, there's only need for a single sperm. But, while the man ejaculates about 100 to 300 million sperm, less than 100,000 make it to the woman's cervix, and only a few hundred will reach the woman's fallopian tubes.

Women are born with all the eggs they will release. However, males will begin producing sperm in early puberty and with age, sperm production and mobility is prone to diminish. This aspect carries a lot of importance. So, can a man actually maximize his odds of producing high-quality sperm that increases your chances of conceiving? Yes. Here are some top health tips that will help your guy to improve his fertility.

#1 Diet matters for men too

The cliché expression known by every one of us "you are what you eat" is 100 percent true. A healthy body will increase the man's chances of producing healthy, mobile sperm. Actual studies point that a diet consisting of high levels of potent antioxidants that are found in fruits and veggies can genuinely restore and support the reproductive system. Studies indicate that the man's diet can seriously affect a couple's ability to conceive.

To be more precise, insufficiency in vitamin A, C, D, E, B12, selenium, and zinc can genuinely lead to lower sperm count and motility. A healthy diet equals healthy sperm, not to mention that the man's sexual performance will be much better. In a nutshell, a nutrient-full diet is crucial for ensuring your man's fertility as well.

#2 Limit workout activities

Athletes who exhaust themselves with strenuous workouts on a regular basis are prone to have a low sperm production. It's true that exercise is crucial for supporting a good health condition, as well as a balanced hormonal output, but in the case of exhaustion, the body's energy is directed toward helping the body in recovering from fatigue. That indeed inhibits natural testosterone levels from being produced.

#3 Avoid chronic stress

Chronic stress will imminently have an adverse influence on the man's sperm production. Typically, emotional and psychological stress will interfere with the man's testosterone production which is necessary for healthy sperm release. To be more precise, infertility-related stress will have a significant negative impact on both partners, not to mention their relationship. I will provide you with a bunch of tips on how to limit stress when trying to conceive later on in the book.

#4 Have more folate

I already mentioned the crucial significance of folic acid for mothers-to-be. But let's not overlook the dad's job in the whole conception equation. Men require folic acid supplements as well. Studies show us that men who presented lower amounts of folic acid in their diets had different chromosomes in their sperm. When an abnormal sperm fertilizes the egg, the birth may result in miscarriage or birth defects.

To put it roughly, the greater majority of miscarriages that take place in the first trimester occur because of chromosol abnormality. However, this doesn't necessarily mean that your man has to take the same amount of vitamin supplements as you do. But, he should make sure that he has a proper folic acid intake from consuming plenty of veggies, whole grain, and fruits.

#5 Drink less soda

Sodas equal large amounts of sugar are more than harmful to a couples' health. To be more precise, excess intake of sugary drinks will interfere with the man's testosterone production.

#6 Steer clear of lubricants during intercourse

Even though there is still ongoing research that is yet to prove the link between infertility and lubricant use, it is recommended that you avoid using lubricants during intercourse. They seem to have an adverse impact on the quality of the sperm. A positive alternative to commercially-produced lubricants is olive oil, coconut oil, baby oil, or fertility-friendly lubricant.

How to give birth to a healthy child?

As for giving birth to a healthy child, there are plenty of ways for you to do that. I already expanded on the crucial importance of nutrition and diet in a previous chapter about preparing the body for pregnancy. What about the actual process of giving birth to a healthy child? Diet matters in this case too, and the fertility diet I shared with you above will ensure that you accomplish this target as well. Diet, environment and lifestyle choices are crucial for preserving your health as a mother to be, and the health of your future baby. I would like to offer you an example of the way in which your diet can present a crucial impact on the health of your child.

Your baby's brain is composed of fat. Don't be surprised or scared, as this is perfectly normal. As a matter of fact, the human brain features 2/3 fat, besides water, minerals and glucose. I mentioned the crucial significance of including fats in your diet, and now I want to outline that they play an essential role in the construction of your baby's brain structure. In simpler terms, your diet will influence how smart your baby will be during his/her lifetime. Really? Really. Usually, the fats consist of up to 70 percent of the entire process of making new connections between the neurons inside the baby's brain. To put it roughly, more links equal a smarter child.

There is plenty of research and talk concerning the importance of omega 3 fatty acids for fetal development. These can be found in veggies, nuts, organic meat and fish. Typically, this is the fuel that supports the development of the baby's brain and health.

I would like to provide you with another example of the way in which you can increase your probability of conceiving a healthy child. If you didn't know it yet, vitamin D intake is more than essential for genetic regulation. Vitamin D has been proven to prevent autism.

In a nutshell, as a conclusion to this detailed chapter, in the majority of cases I've personally dealt with, couples who considered these practical pieces of advice and tips managed to conceive and are now happily content with their babies and extended family. I know how agonizing it must be for you to try to get pregnant and assume that everything seems to fail. Please take into consideration these aspects, which were proven to be helpful, and see for yourself. A proper diet and nutrition, accompanied by positive lifestyle choices are genuinely beneficial for living a healthy life, not only for becoming pregnant.

Take your time and think about what you have eaten in the last 150 days. Don't be surprised. 150 days is how much it takes for the cells in your body to be replaced. More accurately, every atom in your body is replaced within a certain amount of time. Are those hot dogs and burgers coming back to you now? It is important to comprehend that everything you have put in your mouth in the last 150 days contributed to your present health state. As you long to get pregnant, the expression "you are what you eat" certainly applies to your case, doesn't it?

Improving the quality of the food you eat as you try to get pregnant is primordial. You must make sure that your cells are healthy, and your hormonal production is balanced.

Chapter 5: Understand the Link between Stress and Infertility

In this chapter, you will learn:

- How infertility and stress are related.
- How to overcome infertility stress efficiently.

If you have been attempting to get pregnant for months, then you probably feel angry whenever a friend or relative approaches you to tell you that you need to relax and let nature take its course. You know what I'm referring to, don't you? Still, as unrealistic as it may appear, at first, there seems to be a definite link between stress and infertility. Specialists have determined that stress can lead to infertility in 30 percent of the cases.

You need to comprehend that your body, mind and soul create a whole. If you're stressed out and constantly reminiscing negative emotions and feelings, despairing that you won't manage to get pregnant, all these thoughts can actually be the triggering factors that prevent you from conceiving. Your body is not separated from your thoughts and feelings. On the contrary, the harmful physiological effects stress has on the body can genuinely affect your odds of conception.

From my personal experience, stress is detrimental to us on so many levels, not only when trying to get pregnant. Stress negatively affects your well-being as well.

Let me explain to you what stress does to your body. When you are stressed, the hormone levels of epinephrine and cortisol significantly grow and remain that way during times of chronic stress. This can affect the production of hormones that help you to get pregnant. In the same respect, diminishing stress can also improve proteins inside the uterine lining that play a core role in the process of implantation. Stress reduction can contribute to increasing blood flow to the uterus, which can grow your odds of conception.

Studies conducted in this domain show that 40 percent of the couples that tried to get pregnant did not present any obvious health issue that caused this fact. Therefore, scientists affirm that the stress factor had profoundly detrimental effects on the couple's fertility. It is quite evident if you take a moment to think about it. The lifestyles we have are very stressful – we deal with all kinds of pressure, whether it's at work, at home or in relationships, we seem to be overwhelmed, and always, always on the run.

These charts were distinct a few years ago. Unexplained infertility in couples was estimated at 10 percent at that time, compared to the present when it has reached 40 percent. While our bodies haven't altered in any way, our stressed lifestyles have indeed changed us. Another factor that seems to frighten most women and make them stressed is constantly thinking that the biological clock is ticking, and it's their last chance of conception. I believe that this is the first stage that leads to infertility.

Overcome infertility stress

If you had encountered difficulties conceiving, stress could be the underlying root of your problem. Please take a close look at your life, and acknowledge if stress is a big part of your daily existence or not. Be honest with yourself. I'm not talking about the regular stressful daily outcomes everybody deals with. I refer to chronic, intense stress at work, or trying to cope with more than you should. Whether it is stress related to your infertility – which is sadly quite common in most women, or to other causes, it may be the reason you're lying confused, reading this book, and not knowing why you're not pregnant yet. Cheer up. It will happen.

There is clear evidence suggesting that letting go of stress is very helpful in increasing the odds of conception. You might be saying to yourself that it can't possibly be that simple, aren't you? But it is. Your body reacts to what it goes through on a daily basis: when you don't have time for yourself, and you don't allow yourself to rest and unwind, or when you always torment yourself or your partner with negative thoughts on your infertility issues. Such a behavior actually means that you are unconsciously sabotaging your chances of having a baby. Believe me, I know what I'm talking about. A lot of women have gone through what you're going through. We want to have it all. But we can't. You can't cope with everything at a time. You have to take things slowly, and allow yourself to breathe. Don't force yourself, because your body will respond to that negatively.

Now, let's move on to a couple of tips on how to overcome your stress related to your infertility issues.

#1 Acupuncture

Research in this domain shows that acupuncture may be the key to many infertility problems. Studies developed in Germany, which were published in the journal entitled "Fertility and Sterility", included women who opted for acupuncture before and after the fertilization of the egg. Compared to the other women who didn't benefit from acupuncture treatment, the first group of women was 42.5 percent more prone to becoming pregnant.

Acupuncture seems to be quite effective in decreasing stress and helping women deal with it better, as it helps counterbalance some of the harmful impacts stress has on the mind and body. Keep on reading about acupuncture and its marvelous effects in the following chapter.

#2 Relaxation massage

Another useful alternative might be opting for relaxation massages, which contribute to reducing the body's levels of stress. Research shows that a relaxing massage helps to relieve stress and other health-related problems. What I recommend to every woman reading this book and trying to get pregnant is to take a moment and look into her life and notice the little things that make her stressed and less joyful.

#3 Calming practices

I would also recommend engaging in a calming, soothing practice, or a hobby that keeps your mind calmed and positive. I suggest one of the following habits that can help you reduce stress. You can think of other ideas as well; I'm only suggesting a few.

Keep a detailed journal – Keeping a journal can help you to deal with your emotions better. As you write your feelings and emotions, you will feel freed from them, and thus, you can cope with your depression concerning your infertility much better. I consider this practice quite helpful. Every time I go through negative experiences, when I put it all in writing, somehow I feel released, and I no longer act negatively with people around me. If you don't do something about your negativity, it will imminently affect those around you.

Meditation – Taking some time off your busy schedule to clear your mind through meditation can significantly aid you to relief stress and embrace a peaceful state of mind. Meditation allows you to embrace yourself, accept yourself and cope with your feelings better. Many people associate meditation with religious practices, which is quite a popular misconception. Meditation is simply a method of achieving utter and complete relaxation.

Warm, relaxing baths – Relaxation methods are pretty efficient, as I already said, and having warm baths can help you to relax and unwind from stress.

#4 Plan a vacation – Conceptionmoon

Vacations are all about taking a break, unwinding and letting go of your troubles and worries, isn't it? Why not plan a lovely vacation with your partner, so that you get away from it all and get pregnant? You might be skeptical at first, but from my experience, a lot of couples I've worked with managed to solve that infertility issue when on vacation.

[67]

If you have a demanding job, perhaps other kids at home and other daily problems that combined altogether somehow prevent you from getting fully relaxed, this might be why you're not pregnant yet! Trust me! I talked to a lot of couples who have struggled for months to get pregnant, and after having a beautiful, romantic vacation, guess what happened? You guessed that right. They cured infertility!

I suggest you don't delay it any longer, and consider talking to your partner about this possibility. Think of a vacation destination that makes you feel relaxed and happy and book it without having second thoughts! Whether you wish to go to the mountains, or at the seaside, never mind, as long as you let go of all your negative feelings and just enjoy a relaxing time with your beloved. For a couple of days, forget that you're trying to get pregnant and enjoy spending time with your partner, and revive the romance. If you feel like every time you get together all you're thinking about is getting pregnant, perhaps you need to leave those thoughts behind, and just relax.

Believe it or not, there is actual research that proves the high effectiveness of a nice, relaxing vacation. It's not called conception moon for anything!

5 Seek counseling

Struggling with infertility problems can be quite demanding, emotionally speaking. Complex emotional problems are quite common in couples who cannot succeed to get pregnant.

A friend of mine, Clara, had been trying to get pregnant right after she got married to Nathan. However, their plans seemed not to come to reality, and as months kept passing by, they dreaded the abundance of questions such as "when will we see a little one with you?" and so on, and they had no affirmative answer. As a couple, they were diagnosed with unexplained infertility.

Clara started doing some research in this field and found out that one in seven women deals with infertility at some point in her life. She was astonished when finding out that one in seven women deals with the same problems she had. But when you're trying to conceive and the odds seem to be against you, somehow you feel like you're the only one in that situation.

Overwhelmed by all these negative emotions and feelings, being unable to understand why everyone around her seemed to get pregnant in spite of her, all added up, and it was genuinely too much for her to cope with. After discussing with Nathan, they decided they should opt for counseling as things were standing still and not moving forward, and they felt under the weather most of the times. Somehow, talking to each other about the situation didn't help, as they weren't able to encourage one another. They were unable to explain to one another what is happening, and why they can't begin their own family. They turned to counseling that ought to help them deal with the ambiguity of their situation. And the good news is that it actually did help them. As they freed themselves from all that negativity and unanswered questions they have gathered from them for months, they managed to regain their joy in life and leave stress behind.

Clara stopped blaming herself for not being able to become pregnant. Nathan stopped blaming himself for not being good enough for making their dream come true. After they implemented some healthy lifestyle and dietary changes, continuing with their regular counseling session, Clara and Nathan finally got pregnant, and now, their little girl – Abby – is three years old, and she fills their lives with joy and laughter.

Clara and Nathan, somewhere on the path, have lost one another and got fixed on this single idea of getting pregnant, which they unconsciously associated with negativity and frustration. Their fear regarding the fact that they were dealing with infertility caused a lot of tensions to add up to their relationship. Counseling made them realize that this assimilated tension actually created a more stressful living environment.

It is important to find support while you're trying to get pregnant, and you might be dealing with unexplained infertility. This is most of the times caused by a myriad of different factors, which make the possibility of pregnancy lower.

Counseling can truly help you. Speak to your partner about it. Perhaps freeing you from stress and negative emotions is all you need to get pregnant and expect your baby!

Chapter 6: Alternative Methods for Maximizing Fertility

In this chapter, you will learn:

- How acupuncture can be the key to curing infertility.
- How fertility yoga can help you conceive.

It's no secret that fertility treatments cost a lot of money, somewhere ranging between $10,000 and $20,000. Typically, an in vitro fertilization costs about $12, 400, without mentioning the medicine attached to the procedure. However, if you're yearning to become a mother, why not try some alternative ways of conceiving? Acupuncture, yoga, and complementary therapies are acknowledged as viable alternatives to these costly treatments, which, in plenty of cases, have been proven highly effective. Let's get into this matter.

Acupuncture

Acupuncture is an ancient Chinese practice that uses the stimulation of pressure points to bring balance into a person suffering from a health condition. The most popular method is that of inserting needles into particular parts of the skin. This particular technique was highly used in China and other Asian countries to cure nicotine addiction, a myriad of pains, thyroid conditions, migraines and others.

And, surprising to us, in China, acupuncture has been used in treating infertility for centuries. In this direction, researchers have conducted several studies to prove whether acupuncture is actually useful when treating infertility or not.

Understanding acupuncture

It's important that we understand how it works, and what lies behind the whole concept of acupuncture. First, acupuncture encompasses the presence of an energy force known as chi, which traverses the body on meridians or channels. This energy has a strong influence on every aspect of a person's life – emotional, spiritual, mental and psychical. Yin and yang are two forces that dwell within the chi, and they must be in perfect balance for the best health condition.

When the two paralleled forces are imbalanced, then, several health problems may occur. Experienced acupuncturists insert needles in particular spots for unblocking the chi.

Old Chinese Medicine outlines some patterns for infertility problems in women such as shortage of energy, irregular menstrual cycles, and chronic stress. To be more precise, acupuncture practices for infertility in women concentrate on the heart, kidneys, and liver. First and foremost, the kidneys ensure the body's energy levels, so, curing this area would grow a woman's strength to conceive and nurture a developing fetus. Treating the liver, on the other hand, is supposed to control menstrual flow and diminish the detrimental effects of depression, anxiety disorder and PMS. And lastly, the heart is known to be in strong relation with a person's feelings and emotions, so diminishing stress and facilitating complete relaxation can help with the conception process. When all these areas are taken care of, the woman's menstrual cycles will be regulated, and the egg released by the ovaries will be healthier.

As I already mentioned before, the primary triggering cause of the polycystic ovarian syndrome is hormonal imbalance. PCOS occurs when the woman releases a high level of male hormones, which will lead to a stressing imbalance in her body. Acupuncture techniques will aim at bringing balance and enhancing blood flow to the reproductive organs, the fact that contributes to restoring the proper functioning of the ovaries.

Plus, the improvement of blood circulation will strengthen the endometrium – the lining surrounding the uterus – making it thicker. That will facilitate the fertilization process. And this is not all. Acupuncture can help control thyroid hormones and decrease weight, which are two main factors linked to infertility. Nonetheless, if the woman who wishes to get pregnant suffers from thyroid dysfunctions, the acupuncturist will treat different meridians.

Other important factors are timing and consistency. If you would like to have a better health condition, you should opt for two sessions per week for up to six months. The hormones inside a woman's body can be regulated during her menstrual cycle. This is why acupuncturists suggest at least 12 treatments or three consecutive menstrual cycles. Acupuncture is highly recommended for women who want to opt for in vitro fertilization, and wish to grow their chances of conceiving. According to studies, the perfect timing for this type of treatment is marked by the luteal phase during the menstrual cycle.

Acupuncture can work for men coping with infertility as well. It is highly useful for mean dealing with stress-related infertility, low sperm count, and low sperm quality. In most cases, the acupuncture treatment for men lasts for up to three months.

Yoga

There are numerous types of yoga, and it is a truth universally acknowledged that yoga helps control breathing, improves general health condition and facilitates meditation. Plus, it improves flexibility, strength, and balance.

However, there is more to yoga than what meets the eye. It seems that scientists have recently uncovered that yoga can have a positive influence in dealing with several health conditions such as cardiovascular diseases, poor immune system, and problems of the nervous system. And for you, who are eager to get pregnant, yoga can do wonders as it can genuinely enhance your fertility and improve the right functioning of your reproductive system.

[73]

Even so, you shouldn't expect yoga to treat health conditions such as blocked tubes or cysts, but what will yoga fix is your fertility problems rooted in today's modern malady – stress. It's a marvelous relaxation technique, and, as the majority of women dealing with fertility are angry at their bodies, yoga can aid them to embrace their bodies and feel better about themselves.

Everybody deals with stress on a regular basis, and it's entirely reasonable. But the moment in which fear becomes a big part of your life, it will trigger the appearance of numerous health problems, including infertility, anxiety disorders, cardiovascular diseases, depression, and weakened immune system.

Stress plays a crucial role in the whole infertility equation, and it's tricky. To put it roughly, infertility causes stress, and stress can cause infertility. Are you confused yet? The truth is that infertility-related stress is terrible, and most women who are yearning to become mothers know what I'm referring to. And yoga can help you to cope with that kind of stress.

Yoga could have beneficial effects on your infertility issues if you didn't know that yet. It can and will improve your fertility, preparing your body for pregnancy. Fertility Yoga encompasses a broad range of stretches that present beneficial effects on the reproductive system, in this way growing your fertility. Every posture Fertility Yoga includes supports and adds positive influence on the reproductive and endocrine system. If you consider making the dietary and lifestyle changes I've enumerated in the previous chapter and practice Fertility Yoga as well, you'll be expecting a baby in no time.

The most significant benefit that comes with practicing Fertility Yoga is that it contributes to bringing your hormones back into balance. Additionally, it improves the reproductive system's circulation, while at the same time supporting the body and the immune system. This type of yoga will improve your overall health and wellbeing, and every aspect of your life. You will feel reimbursed with positive energy.

In spite of the fact that there is still ongoing research concerning the effects yoga has on couple's fertility, the truth is that you can diminish your body's stress response by practicing yoga. This way, you can grow your chances of conceiving. There have been several studies conducted in this area. For example, a study carried out on infertile individuals who practiced yoga specifically designed for decreasing stress reflected a fertility boost of up to 35 percent.

And for those of you who are yearning to become parents, yoga will help you get rid of all that stress and guilt you might be feeling that is eating you from the inside out.

A study indicates that people who practiced yoga on a regular basis experienced higher levels of gamma-aminobutyric acid – GABA, compared to those who didn't practice yoga. This hormone is crucial because it aims at regulating the mood, and when the levels are low, we are prone to suffering from depression and anxiety, which leads to infertility.

The best yoga practices for eager parents to be are Hatha and Anasura yoga styles, which successfully reduce stress.

Mind/Body techniques

The research developed concerning the effectiveness of mind and body techniques presented promising results. During techniques such as guided imagery, cognitive behavioral therapy or deep breathing, the patient helps turn negative thoughts into positive ones. The majority of couples dealing with infertility cope with chronic stress and these techniques are helpful in this direction. However, in most cases, they ought to be combined with lifestyle modifications, wholesome diet, and counseling for best results. The fact is that each couple is different, and there's a combination of methods that will work for every particular patient.

Chapter 7: The Importance of Detoxifying Your Body

In this chapter, you will learn:

- The benefits of detoxifying your body.
- Basic tips on a healthy body detox.

A healthy body is a key to conceiving a child. That is why you need to take the time to prepare for conception while at the same time increasing the chances of getting pregnant. Thus, I heartedly recommend to you to detoxify your body from all the harmful toxins that may affect your fertility and, this way, you will have a better chance to start a healthy lifestyle for the sake of your newborn.

Our bodies can cope with toxins, to some extent. But, nowadays, we are regularly exposed to toxins, and this has a harmful impact on us. As you're preparing for pregnancy, you might be taking all sorts of herbal supplements, engaging in calming Yoga practices or eating clean. Still, there might be harmful toxins underlying in your body. Detoxifying your body will contribute to getting your hormones into balance and reinvigorating your health condition.

I had a friend to whom I always lectured about the importance of a healthy diet and so on. Still, my talks seemed to reach no place, as she kept on ignoring me. Until she decided she wanted to get pregnant, and told me how she wanted to start fresh. I congratulated her for her wise choice, and I heartedly recommend you do the same. My friend managed to get pregnant, and is now a happy mother of a two-year-old, Markus.

Detoxifying your body can only have beneficial impacts on your chances of getting pregnant and, afterward, on growing a healthy baby inside of you. Because of the abundance of harmful toxins, most babies are, unfortunately, born pre-polluted. To put it roughly, mothers will implement part of the toxins that lie in their bodies into their growing infants. You won't be happy to find this out, of course. The math is simple. Toxins will keep on harming your child as he grows up, but you can diminish the early exposure to these toxins by considering to take a range of detoxifying steps.

Don't get me wrong. Detoxifying your body doesn't necessarily imply staying on a strict diet, fasting and drinking only carrot and beet juices. While the human body is naturally equipped with the ability to detoxify itself, because we are daily exposed to various toxins, it might need a little help. So, I recommend you try the following tips on detoxifying your body naturally and being perfectly healthy so that you can get pregnant and start expecting a baby!

#1 Drink lemon water

This is an easy, cost-effective habit, which will bring you a myriad of health benefits. Add ½ the juice of a lemon to one quart of water and it will contribute to detoxifying your liver. Lemons are filled with antioxidants and nutrients as well, boosting your metabolism.

#2 Take detoxifying baths

Allow me to present to you the great benefits that come with detox baths. Typically, they are simple baths, to which you add Epsom salts or baking soda, and that will help your body to release the unwanted toxins. Taking detox baths will also contribute to regulating the production of enzymes in the body. Also, they help to reduce inflammation, while at the same time improving the body's ability to remove harmful toxins. Detox baths are also popular for helping you cope with stress better. In order to prepare a great detox bath, you can use Epsom salts (two cups to one bathtub) or even baking soda (four cups to one tub of water). Another option would be using your favorite essential oil – 10 drops mixed with a carrier oil (coconut oil or jojoba oil). Add this particular combo to your regular bath and enjoy the scent and its excellent benefits.

#3 Introduce herbs with cleansing properties

Drinking dandelion tea or including flaxseeds in your diet can also aid you to eliminate all those harmful toxins in your body.

#4 Hit the sauna

Hitting the sauna once in a while can help you restore skin elimination. More accurately, it will help your body remove the toxins, kill the germs, and boost your metabolism. You can also use a more modern approach: infrared saunas. They use lower temperatures (up to 130°F), but they are usually taken for a longer period. The studies have revealed that this is better than the traditional sauna because it promotes fat sweat, thus helping you get rid of the harmful toxins stored in fat. Regular saunas only stimulate water sweat, where the toxins are not that many. An infrared sauna can help you eliminate uric acid, cholesterol, sodium, cadmium, mercury and other heavy metals, ammonia and sulfuric acid. Typically, infrared saunas are acknowledged to be one of the best yet safest ways to promote full detoxification and increase your overall health condition. For the mother to be, they are an excellent way to eliminate harmful toxins in the body.

#5 Opt for organic beauty products

The exposure to beauty products that are filled with chemicals can harm your health immensely. Thus, I recommend you limit your use of products that aren't organic, and consider opting for natural ones.

Chapter 8: Emotional Problems Fertility-Challenged Women Go Through

In this chapter, you will learn:

- How to conquer your emotional challenges.
- That you are not alone in your struggle.
- That you can overcome these challenges with proper support.
- How to overcome the emotional stress of experiencing a miscarriage.

Fertility-challenged women start their journey towards motherhood with a sole purpose in their mind, which is that of giving birth to a baby. Their vision is clear, knowing that having a baby is their purpose in life, and they get excited solely at the thought of getting pregnant. As soon as you try to conceive, and you see that nothing happens, you begin to worry, and as months pass by, you become more and more stressed and emotionally-charged. Thus, I want to tell you how to deal with the emotional challenges infertility makes you go through.

#1 Acquiring emotional balance

To you, the woman who's trying to get pregnant, it's no secret that your infertility problems have made you go through a roller coaster of negative emotions and feelings. You might feel like you wish to give it all up at times. But what you need to know is that you should aim at acquiring emotional balance, and keeping your feelings in control. This is the key.

I understand how you change your mood every two days. One day you're happy that you're doing all it takes to get pregnant and that sooner you'll be telling your partner that you're expecting, and the next day you feel like you wish to give it all up because there are no clear answers to your problem.

Don't give up, you need to be powerful and believe in yourself. And, as you do everything that stays in your power to get pregnant, this will eventually happen, and you'll feel like a new person. Meditation and yoga practices have helped a lot of women struggling with infertility.

#2 Don't let go of your sense of humor and joy of life

As you start your journey towards getting pregnant, in the beginning, you will feel reinvigorated and positive about having a baby. However, as time passes by, and you're still not pregnant, life isn't funny or enjoyable anymore. You lose your wish to laugh at yourself. And there's nothing more frustrating to a woman who yearns to become a mother than hearing all sorts of jokes such as "I can barely sleep at night because of my children, I can give them to you if you want!"

My advice is not to let this experience darken your life; don't let go of your sense of humor and joy of life. You need to be positive and be thankful for being alive and for having your partner beside you.

#3 Maintain your self-identity

A lot of women facing infertility will lose their sense of identity on the road. I'm not talking about getting physically older. I'm referring to the emotional struggle you are going through. Don't let that happen. Don't let infertility destroy your identity and, please, recapture the joy that you used to feel each time you went for a walk or spent time with your partner. You need to embrace your body and accept yourself.

#4 Forgive your body

Every woman who tried to have a baby and didn't succeed knows what I'm talking about. Please stop blaming your body. You need to regain your self-worth and forgive your body for not getting pregnant, because, on a subconscious level, you are blaming it for your unhappiness. Instead, take care of your body, nurture it and leave negativity behind.

[80]

#5 Stop blaming

I want to challenge you to stop blaming yourself, or your partner for your lack of success in getting pregnant. This is quite a challenge, isn't it? Please stop putting the blame on any of you two; a lot of couples have managed to get pregnant after years, and I'm referring to real people here. You're not the only couple facing this problem. As long as you aim at stopping the continuous blame, accepting yourself, and embracing a positive attitude towards your reality, you'll manage to regain your identity and self-worth.

How to overcome emotional stress if you've had a miscarriage in the past?

Now, I would like to address those women who have gone through the immense pain of losing a baby through miscarriage. I know you find it almost impossible to get over your loss. But, that's normal, and it's ok. Pregnancy loss is a devastating experience, and, in the position of the mother you are entitled to grieve for your baby. All the anticipation and preparation that begins from the second you have found out about your pregnancy becomes so painful once you realize that he/she is no longer living inside of you.

Most women feel guilt and anger directed towards their own bodies. But, you have to remember that miscarriages happen naturally, and they're nobody's fault. Try not to direct your negativity towards your partner, because, even though you may think that he is not going through the same emotional stress as you are, he actually is. Other women may fall into anxiousness and may feel as if they were never meant to become mothers. What I wish to outline is that regardless of the feelings you are experiencing – and I know they are hurting you – you must allow them to exist and accept them. You have the right to feel them because you have lost your unborn baby.

[81]

If you and your partner encounter difficulties in communicating, that is ok too. Just give each other time to mourn. Still, it's important that you express the emotions you are feeling to each other, and help one another go through this episode from your lives. You probably observed the tendency to isolate yourself from your partner. If you realize that it has become a stressing issue, address your problem to a specialist. What you further need to comprehend is that people mourn differently, so what seems to you like lack of love and consideration may not be that to a different individual. Plus, the mother experiences the miscarriage differently, as she was the one who was carrying the baby inside of her. Don't blame your partner for not feeling the same as you do.

Everyone grieves differently

I want to outline that everyone grieves in his/her own way. Please do comprehend that grieving is an individual experience. Your mindset and state of being will depend on a broad range of distinguishing factors such as your personality, life experience, nature of the loss, etc. Plus, most importantly, you should recognize that grieving takes time – healing is part of an elaborate, individual process. You cannot force it, nor can you hurry it, so that you get over your suffering fast and get it over with. As much as it hurts, try to embrace your feelings.

Many parents I've talked to have reported feeling better after weeks while others after months. However, in spite of that, one golden rule does apply in all cases – be patient with yourself, and with your partner as well.

Many people are told or they assume that by ignoring the pain, it will go away. I don't reckon this approach being helpful to any of the persons in this dark scenario. Trying to ignore the pain will make it surface in the long term. The healing process imminently implies dealing with the grief, and facing it, even though it seems like the most difficult thing to do.

If you hear people telling you over and over again that you need to be strong, don't feel like that's something you must do. Feeling anxious, frightened and lonely is normal – you needn't feel that you have to prove anyone your inner strength, especially at such a point in your life. A quite common reaction is crying, but many parents don't seem to find the power within them to cry. That doesn't mean your baby wasn't important to you, and that you didn't love him/her with all your heart. People who don't typically cry experience pain differently, and that's entirely normal, and you shouldn't feel that you have to cry your eyes out to prove someone you loved your baby. Remember, you don't owe anyone anything.

Coping with grief when you feel down

At this unique stage in your life, you should focus on you – you needn't direct your attention towards the way in which your friend and family convey your situation, or determine them to feel sorry for you or anything like that. Something I say to every woman who deals with miscarriage is – take care of yourself. A major loss such as a miscarriage may deplete your energy and emotional reserve, leaving you feeling empty. Watching after your emotional and physical needs will enable you to go through this experience, and become a stronger version of yourself.

Face your feelings. While you may aim at suppressing your grief, assuming that this is the way to go through it, the truth is that you cannot keep avoiding it forever. Avoidance is an unconscious mechanism of defense you might be tempted to embrace, but it's a trap. Healing imminently implies acknowledging the pain. Avoiding your feelings of loss and suffering, and dismissing them as if they weren't even there, will only prolong the pain, making it an important part of your life and marriage. Unresolved grief leads to severe complications such as prolonged depression, anxiety, and health problems.

[83]

Express your feelings. You shouldn't feel afraid or hesitant towards expressing the feelings that feature this difficult phase in your life. Settle what works best for you. You could try writing about your experience in a journal, writing a letter, or talking about what you're facing with your partner, a friend, or a specialist.

Look after your physical health. Your mind and body are linked, and everything you experience has a substantial impact on your body as well. Combat stress and negativity by eating right, and engaging in plenty of exercises – healthy habits are good for you. Pursue them, as opposed to using sleeping pills or other artificial methods of boosting your mood, which, in the long term, will do you more harm than good.

Don't permit anyone to tell you how you should be feeling. When you go through something such as a miscarriage, many people will come to you offering you advice. Remember, you shouldn't feel embarrassed, or judged by their input. You needn't embrace every piece of advice you receive, and you shouldn't feel like you owe someone something.

Know that you're not alone. If you don't have an answer to many of your questions, you should find out that the vast majority of stillborn cases and miscarriages are triggered by external causes. And most importantly, it's not your fault. Period. It happened, but you're not the one to blame. Also, remember that experiencing a miscarriage doesn't mean that you're likely to experience another one. Nearly half of the women have such an incident at some point in their lives. Hence, you're not the only woman in this position. That should encourage you to move on, and embrace the next phase in your life.

Will a miscarriage affect my ability to give birth to a healthy child?

Typically, you should no longer be thinking about this, because a miscarriage doesn't necessarily imply that you won't be able to have a healthy child in the future. It doesn't mean that you'll experience the same problems with the next pregnancy. Make sure you surpass this phase of your life, embrace your body and accept yourself. If you are still dealing with anxiety and stress related to pregnancy, it is not recommended to try conceiving until you have surpassed this phase. If you won't be able to have a baby soon after the miscarriage, you will be even sadder and depressed. Just take a break for and try to accept the situation.

Typically, miscarriage is recognized as a one-time occurrence, and the greater majority of women who go through it will develop a healthy pregnancy afterward. Only a small percentage of women – namely 1 percent – will experience multiple miscarriages. While there's nothing left for you to do in order to prevent a miscarriage, pursuing a healthy lifestyle, and making healthy decisions for you and your future baby's wellbeing is primordial.

Best Practices and Common Mistakes

Do's

- **Think positively**. When dealing with infertility, it might be difficult to remain cheerful and positive, but you need to do your best because stress can be one of the triggering factors preventing you from conceiving.

- **Take proper care of your body.** As I tried to point out throughout the book, I genuinely want you to understand that you need to take care of your body. Make healthy, positive life decisions, and alter those habits that hurt your health. These are the first actions you need to take when conceiving: eating clean and trying to stay healthy. Remember this – your body cannot handle the challenge of pregnancy if it's not properly equipped.

Don'ts

- **Don't let infertility destroy your identity.** As you try to get pregnant, infertility seems to define you, and you no longer find pleasure and joy in your hobbies. Don't let it affect you, try counseling or discussing your fears with someone so that you can overcome them positively.

- **Don't let your infertility issues separate you from your partner.** A lot of couples who struggle with infertility end up separating from one another. As frustration keeps adding up, they unconsciously blame each other or themselves, and the state of the relationship decays. This will only lower your chances of getting pregnant, and will hurt the one you actually love. Don't let that happen.

[86]

Conclusion

I hope that, after having gone trough this book, you realize how important it is to remain positive and think of your purpose during all this process of trying to conceive. I know how badly you yearn to be a mother, and I understand you because I've been there too. I've heard the stories of other parents, just like you, who were mothers, but lacked a baby. And I sincerely trust that the advice and information included in this book will help you reach your goal. Your lifestyle choices are more important than you might believe. I want you to understand that.

I know that having a baby is one of the biggest decisions we make in our lives, and I understand how frustrating it is for you to deal with infertility, as you and your partner are prepared to take this step forward. I know.

There are thousands of couples, just like you, that have tried to get pregnant for months and even years, and eventually succeeded. As soon as you realize that you're not the only one struggling with this problem, I believe you'll feel better.

Your dreams of becoming a mother will become a reality in your life. But you have to take proper care of your body, nourish it and love it honestly and offer it a good diet. Listen to its reactions because it knows what's best for you. Don't let yourself become overwhelmed with stress and negativity. Find support in your partner, or if not, counseling can be a positive idea. I believe you'll make the right choices, after reading this book, and you'll be holding your perfect baby in your arms sooner than you might be expecting! I wish you all the best in the world. Take care and don't lose your faith! It will happen!

Intermittent Fasting:

Lose Fat Fast - Fasting, Dieting, Adrenal Reset & Flexible Ketogenic Diet

Introduction

We have always been told throughout these years that we should start our days by having a healthy breakfast, for losing weight. This is because the breakfast will boost your metabolism for starting the day. This reminds me of an old saying - "Have your breakfast like a king, your lunch like a prince and have your dinner like a pauper." But we don't know how true it is.

The next thing we hear is that if you want to lose your weight, have several meals in small quantities throughout the day rather than having three. This will help in keeping your metabolism at optimum levels throughout the day. And again, we don't know how true it is.

What you're going to read next will turn it on its head. You're going to see how intermittent fasting helps you lose weight rather than having multiple small meals throughout the day at certain times. If your main goal is to lose weight in a safe and healthy manner, this is the book for you, and I assure you that you will not regret it.

For people who are trying to stabilize their weights by following all the diets, this book can be a turnaround. Many people blame their genes for being overweight, and they say that it runs in their family, but it is wrong. Even for such people, fasting can show amazing results. But you need to know which type of fasting works best for you.

You can find balance in your life with the help of fasting. Compared to dieting, fasting is easier and more effective, and after setting the routine once, it is not hard to incorporate it into your daily life. This book also helps you to decide the best-suited intermittent fasting system, which you can practice in your day-to-day life. Once you get used to it, you can get rid of constipation and digestion problems, as your body will get a chance to heal. People usually blame it on slow metabolism,

[89]

and it is not right. The problems arise due to their eating habits. Try doing it for a long time, and your body will definitely stay healthy. When you take care of your body, it may give you a bonus of living a longer life.

You might have heard about the fad diets: The all fat, no fat, gluten-free eating, raw veggies no dressing, six small meals, cabbage soup have already proven to help people lose weight fast.

What if I tell you that the answer for improving body composition, losing weight and feeling better is not through dieting but by occasionally skipping meals? For some people, fasting for a longer period of time (14-36 hours, usually), without taking any calories, might not be as hard as they think it would be. Technically, we fast every day, and it is called sleeping. Intermittent fasting is nothing but extending the period we fast by slightly being more conscious of your eating habits overall. But, will it be right for you? And which is the best-suited method?

Chapter 1: The Science of Fasting

Earlier, since the 1930s, scientists have been researching about the benefits of reducing the calorie intake by skipping meals. An American scientist from that time discovered that mice live healthier and longer lives by reducing the calories they take. In recent studies, researchers and scientists have found the same in monkeys, roundworms and fruit flies. The studies have also proved that by decreasing the calorie intake by 30% to 40% can significantly extend the lifespan by 30% or more. The risks of many common diseases can be reduced by limiting the food intake. Some people believe that fasting increases the responsiveness of the body to insulin. The feelings of food craving and hunger can be controlled, as insulin regulates blood sugar.

In this book, we will discuss the five most commonly used intermittent fasting methods, and you can take advantage of their benefits. But keep in mind that different methods produce different results for different people. Experts say that if you force yourself to practice a certain method, it won't work. You should choose the right method, which makes your life easier. Not choosing the correct method will make your fasting benefits short lived.

You should know the first step for getting started. Every method will have guidelines of its own for what to eat in your "feeding" phase and the duration to fast. In the next topic, you can find the most popular methods for fasting and the basics on their working. Please note that not everyone can practice intermittent fasting. People having health conditions should visit their doctor before making changes in their usual routine. You should note that the lifestyle and personal goals of a person would be the key factors for choosing the correct fasting method.

Chapter 2: Common weight loss problems/reasons

If you are on a weight loss journey, it is important that you be prepared to face some of the commonly occurring weight loss problems. Here is a list of some the most common weight loss problems and the reasons why some people find it hard to lose weight:

1. Food cravings

Craving for certain foods is different from experiencing hunger. Most weight loss diets involve people staying away from certain foods that are considered unhealthy. Be it chocolates, ice creams, sweets, cheese or snacks rich in carbs like crisps or potato chips, these are the kinds of food that are usually delicious and tasty, and which people indulge in to satisfy their palate. These are the kinds of food people eat even when they are not hungry. These foods may satisfy one's palate, but it is very difficult to burn off the calories accumulated by binging on them. Burning off such calories requires rigorous workouts, which cannot be easily accommodated in your daily schedule. If you have a sweet tooth, it is much harder for you to stay away from these foods.

2. No time for exercise

If you are one of those people who work for long hours and find it difficult to balance family and social life with work, you will most likely find it difficult to lose weight too. The reason is simple: you are so busy with your work and family obligations that you won't find time to work out, even at home. You will find it difficult to fit in a workout regimen in your daily schedule, which means that you will most likely keep putting on pounds and do nothing to burn them off. With almost all kinds of jobholders working for longer hours to meet the demands of their industry and to withstand competition, that's the case with most of them.

3. Dining out at restaurants

Dining out with your family or friends at a restaurant creates a happy social atmosphere, which makes it difficult for you to say no to the not-so-healthy food offered to you. Especially, if your work requires you to travel a lot, you won't find the time and resources to cook for yourself, which means you will be frequenting restaurants or other food places for your daily food.

4. Being lethargic

When you are on a strict diet, your energy levels might get lowered, making you feel lethargic. Especially in the afternoons, you might feel extremely lethargic and too tired to perform any kind of physical activities. When you are low on energy, you will likely give into temptations and start eating junk food to feel energized again.

5. Plateaus

Some people will find it hard to lose weight even after sticking to a strict diet plan. The reason is that low-diet plans tend to slow down your rate of metabolism, making your body go into the 'starvation mode.' So, instead of burning off all the accumulated fat into energy, there will be a reduction in the total energy expenditure of your body.

6. Depression

People taking anti-depressants experience weight gain, so if you are taking such pills, don't be surprised to see that you've gained anywhere from 5 to 15 pounds. Even if you're not on anti-depressants, it is found that there is a correlation between feeling depressed and gaining weight. One of the recent studies found that people who suffer from the feelings of loneliness and sadness tend to put on weight more quickly when compared to others who show fewer signs of depression. People suffering from depression might find solace in eating comfort foods like chocolates or cakes that are high in fat. Or they might simply lose interest in physical or healthy activities which results in them bulking up on pounds. Thus, when people visit doctors complaining of weight gain, most doctors look for the symptoms of depression or the medications they've been taking. Such medicines have a substantial effect on the appetite and metabolism of an individual. Even if the pill makes an individual feel better, they may result in weight gain because of the person regaining his/her appetite.

7. Slower gut

If your bowel movements are slow and experience similar issues related to your gut, they could be one of the reasons for your weight gain. Generally, a healthy human being experiences a bowel movement an hour or so after taking a meal. Having a bowel movement even for once or twice every day is considered healthy. Having irregular bowel movements can be correlated to weight gain. Irregularity in the bowel movements is often caused because of dehydration, the absence of the required amount of gut flora, low fiber intake or taking certain medications.

8. Malnutrition

If you are deficient in minerals like iron, magnesium or in vitamins like vitamin D, it may result in you feeling low on energy. When you feel tired because of malnutrition, you might feel like compensating the low energy levels with foods like sweets, chocolate, coffee or simple carbohydrates. Or you might feel too weak or tired to work out, which ultimately leads to you putting on weight.

9. Healthy appetite

Having a healthy appetite means you have to constantly look at what you are eating. It's no fun trying to lose weight when one has a healthy appetite in general. Even if you think of having only a handful of your favorite (junk) food here and there, see if you are actually being honest with yourself. When you say to yourself 'I am going to have just a cup of chocolate milkshake,' are you really going to drink only a cupful? It is because; drinking glasses, in general, have the capacity of holding as many as three cups. When you keep having a glassful of it here and there, it won't be long before all of the calories add up to fat.

10. Genes do play a part

You might have inherited your tendency to put on weight easily from your parents. Also, studies have shown that women who gained a lot of weight during pregnancy are more likely to give birth to overweight babies. For the baby, the weight issue might continue even into adulthood.

11. Alcohol Consumption

The term 'beer belly' explains it all. Consuming alcohol regularly will result in an overdose of calories, which results in the building up of fat, especially in the abdomen. Such beer bellies are more prevalent in men than in women. If you consume a single glass of wine (5 Oz), you are consuming 120 calories. If you drink a glass of cocktail, you are consuming anywhere between 300 and 400 calories. If you are a habitual drinker, you need to lose the habit if you want to lose weight.

12. Lack of enough sleep

You won't eat when you are asleep, isn't it? Also, sleep deprivation may result in the increase of the levels of the stress hormone 'cortisol,' which in turn results in an increased appetite. So, ensure that you get at least seven hours of sleep every day.

13. Thyroid disorder

Some people have a hard time losing weight because of hormone problems related to the thyroid gland. Hypothyroidism (decreased production of the Thyroid hormone) will result in the piling up of pounds, which become stubborn and tend to stay on forever.

14. Stress

Stress is one of the many factors that contribute to weight gain. If you are stressed out, cortisol is released by your body, which as mentioned earlier, results in an increased appetite.

15. Not eating healthy

Most people think they are following a healthy diet plan, when in reality; the food they eat may not be as healthy as they think. Even people who don't follow a healthy diet plan think what they eat is not unhealthy.

16. Not chewing your food properly

Yes, you heard it right. The process of digestion starts in the mouth, and when you chew your food into liquid, you are aiding the process of digestion, and better digestion can be correlated with weight loss.

17. Working out the wrong way

Every kind of exercise burns calories, but you need to decide on what kind of exercise suits your diet. Doing cardio may not necessarily go well with certain types of diets, while weight training may be necessary for a diet to work for you. You need to equip yourself with the knowledge of what kind of workout suits your diet plan.

18. Paying too much attention to the scale

Most people tend to focus on their weight scale readings to measure their progress. Even if you lose five pounds, your weight may remain the same because of the gain of five pounds of water. So, you need to focus on the fat content of your body instead of focusing on measuring your weight.

19. Lack of consistency

Being consistent while following a diet plan is the key to lose weight. But most people tend to get impatient when they don't see immediate results and get demotivated from proceeding any further. The energy and fervor to follow a diet plan should be maintained for a long time if you want to see a change in your weight.

20. Thinking exercise alone would do the trick

Most people have this misconception that they can lose weight if they exercise, without paying any attention to what they eat. You need to remember that you need to make your body undergo a lot of strain to burn even a small amount of calories. So, the easiest way to keep a check on the calories is to follow a diet plan along with the exercise regimen.

21. Relying on cardio alone

It is a fact that cardio helps in burning calories, but if you keep on practicing cardio without ever lifting even a pound of weight, you are missing the most effective method to lose weight and build strength. By lifting weights, you not only strengthen your joints but also increase the rate of metabolism and muscle mass.

Thus, you need to take a look at all the above factors and decide on where you are lacking in your weight loss endeavors.

Chapter 3. Intermittent Fasting Vs. Crash Dieting

Intermittent Fasting

Intermittent fasting or aggressive dieting is not exactly a diet plan, but a pattern of eating which requires an individual to continuously alternate between eating and fasting.

It is not a diet plan in that it does not specify what foods you need to eat and what foods you need to avoid. It just says *when* you need to eat your food and when you shouldn't. Methods of intermittent fasting involve splitting up of the days of the week into periods alternating between eating and fasting.

We fast every day unknowingly when we go to sleep every day. In intermittent fasting, you just extend the fast for a few more hours. This can be done if you skip your breakfast in the mornings and have your first and last meals at noon and 8 pm respectively.

Let us suppose you sleep for seven hours a day. That could be considered seven hours of fasting. Then with intermittent fasting, you are extending the fast to sixteen hours by skipping breakfast. By following this plan, you are giving a 16-hour gap between your meals, and you consume all your required calories during an eight-hour feeding window.

This is not the only method of intermittent fasting, there are several others proposed by renowned dieticians. Intermittent fasting may seem like a hard thing to do, but in reality, it is relatively easy when compared to the strict diet plans people follow. The fast may seem like it drains energy out of the body, but most people who went ahead with the fasting reported to have felt better and more energized. And remember that you can support the fast by drinking black coffee. Which also suppresses hunger and cravings and at the same time make you feel more energized during your fast.

One of the issues you might face during intermittent fasting is hunger, which will not be that of a problem in the later stages of the fast. As your body gets used to not having food for longer periods of time, hunger will become a less of an issue. During the fast, you are not supposed to consume any solid food, but fluids like water and non-caloric beverages can be consumed. Also, you can drink a bit of coffee or tea during that period. In some methods, like the Warrior Diet, of intermittent fasting, the individual may be allowed to consume foods of low caloric value during the fast.

Crash Dieting and its issues

Another popular form of dieting is crash dieting, which involves an individual severely restricting his/her food intake. In this diet, the individual is supposed to restrict his/her intake of calories so much that they usually starve themselves to meet the diet's protocol. So, technically speaking, crash diet regimens promise weight loss to its customers, provide that they starve themselves for days or weeks. There are many disadvantages to this type of diet plan, even though they may produce substantial results. When it comes to crash dieting, you need a pay a very high price for losing weight. Here are some issues that may arise when you go on a crash diet.

- Following the crash diet does burn fat, but it also results in the loss of muscle, which in turns results in the loss of overall strength of your body.
- This kind of diet will most likely result in nutritional deficiency. Your body requires nutrition for the optimal functioning of various organs and hormonal balance. But when you crash diet, you are depriving your body of essential nutrients, fats, and proteins over a long period of time, which may spell disaster on your overall health. If you are consuming anywhere less than 1200 calories, you need to be put on medical supervision. But crash dieters take the risk of doing the same in their own homes, away from medical settings and monitoring.

- Complications like seizures, unconsciousness, low blood sugar levels; hair loss and even organ failure are associated with extremely low-calorie intake. So, it is important that you keep a check on how you are feeling both mentally and physically while being on a crash diet.
- Your body doesn't allow change easily, which is evident by the fact that it exhibits 'homeostasis, a process which involves the body fighting against change. The degree with which it fights the change is directly proportional to the degree of the change. One of the ways your body tries to achieve homeostasis is by reducing the output of the sympathetic nervous system. This will, in turn, result in the slowing down of the thought process, increased irritability, extreme tiredness and loss of muscle tone.
- Crash dieting will also result in the decrease of the production of sex hormones, which results in the lowering of sex drive and libido.
- A hormone called 'ghrelin' gets prominently released when the body undergoes crash diet. This is the hormone responsible for triggering the feeling of 'hunger.' It means that, when you finally stop being on the crash diet, you will feel hungrier and are likely to binge on food, in what they call the 'rebound' period. This will ultimately result in weight gain again.
- Another undesired effect of crash dieting is the skin becoming loose. If you lose weight quickly over a very short period of time, your skin will have no time to recover and regain its elasticity.

The philosophy of crash dieting in itself doesn't offer anything healthy or good. All it teaches is that you can lose weight if you starve yourselves and doesn't touch upon the subject of healthy habits and balanced diet.

Most of the patients of anorexia or binge eating will have undergone crash dieting at one point or another.

Benefits of intermittent fasting

Now that you have seen the issues of crash dieting, you need to learn how intermittent fasting is different from crash dieting. Here are the benefits of intermittent fasting:

Cellular repair

Your body cleanses and detoxifies itself all day long of the wastes and toxins that enter its system. Cells in our body constantly take part in cellular processes, because of which individual cells, especially the mitochondria might become worn out. Our body sees that such worn out cells are constantly replaced, so as to not cause any disturbance in the cell processes. Extremely low-calorie intake greatly hinders the cell-replacing activity, which is the case with crash dieting. But, even if you are eating food continuously without giving much gap in between the meals, you are not giving time for your body cells to repair themselves. With intermittent fasting, you give enough time for your cells to repair, cleanse and detoxify themselves.

Hormone balance

Intermittent fasting or fasting, in general, has a multifaceted effect on hormones. The levels of human growth hormone get dramatically impacted by fasting. Intermittent fasting in particular results in an increase of the human growth hormone, which aids in the faster growth and repair of muscles. An increase in the hormone also builds endurance. Another important hormone that is hugely impacted by intermittent fasting is insulin. Sometimes when insulin knocks the door of a cell for delivering a package of glucose (energy), the cell ignores it in a condition of what is called 'insulin resistance.' Insulin resistance is one of the contributing factors of most diseases that become chronic over time. Intermittent fasting, when combined with the right workout regimen helps in normalizing the sensitivity of cells towards insulin. Intermittent fasting also helps in normalizing the levels of hormones like leptin (responsible for storing fat) and ghrelin (responsible for initiating hunger). Let us see how leptin regulates the storage of fat. When fat cells accumulate such that the levels of body fat become sufficient for the proper functioning of the body, they release leptin, which takes up the responsibility of informing the brain that it needs to stop producing hunger signals. Studies have shown that people who are obese or overweight usually possess higher levels of leptin. Even though their bodies produce high levels of leptin, they feel hungry and so eat more than required. What actually happens is that, even though leptin yells at the brain that it needs to stop being hungry, the brain will lend a deaf ear to its pleas. The reason is the same as that of insulin resistance; when the brain gets consistently exposed to higher levels of leptin, it loses sensitivity to the hormone's signals. When an individual undergoes intermittent fasting, it provides the brain with an opportunity to hear out what leptin is trying to say.

Weight Loss

In order to understand how intermittent fasting helps in weight loss, you need to know how the body utilizes stored fat. When we consume food, the natural sugars present in it get converted into energy. But when these sugars are in excess and aren't in immediate requirement by the body, the liver stores them in the form of glycogen. When glycogen gets stored to a maximum extent, the energy is stored as fat by the body. Whenever the body needs energy, it will first turn to the glycogen stores. Burning of the glycogen supply requires anywhere between six to eight hours. The body will start burning the fat stored in the fat cells only after depleting the glycogen levels of the liver.

So, when you keep on eating food all day long, or even consume three meals every day, it doesn't give the body an opportunity to burn and utilize the fat reserves. But when you wait longer hours between having meals, it gives the body an opportunity to burn the fat stored in the fat cells.

Anti-aging benefit

Research has shown that intermittent fasting helps in the slowing down of cellular aging. A team of researchers found that when animals suffering from brain related conditions like Alzheimer were made to fast intermittently, they showed a reduction in the brain impairment. They also found that animals undergoing intermittent fasting maintained a leaner muscle mass even as they got older. When the same kinds of experiments were carried out on humans, it was found that intermittent fasting had the same effects on them too.

Thus, aggressive dieting or intermittent fasting is always advantageous, healthier and risk-free when compared to crash dieting.

Chapter 4: Common Intermittent Fasting Diets

Intermittent Fasting: 5 Methods

1. Leangains

Started by: Martain Berkhan

Best suited for: People working out who intended to build muscle and lose body fat.

How It Works: Fast for 16 to 14 hours, for men and women respectively, every day. Now for the remaining 8 to 10 hours, you should "feed." When you are fasting, you're not allowed to consume any calories. You can actually have calorie-free food like sugar-free gum, diet soda, calorie-free sweetness, black coffee, etc. Most of the people practicing this find it easier to fast during the night and breaking the fast roughly after 6 hours after waking. Any person can adapt to this schedule in his lifestyle, and it is very important to maintain the feeding window consistently. If the consistency is not maintained, the hormones can get inoperative, and this will make it hard to continue with the program.

The food you have and the time you eat when feeding will depend on workout time. You should have more carbs on the days you work out, instead of having fat. You should increase your fat intake during your rest days. You should have a good amount of protein every day, and it varies from person to person depending on their activity levels, age, gender, body fat and goals. Irrespective of your program, the majority of your calories should come from whole and unprocessed foods. On a busy day, where you won't have time for a meal, you can actually have a meal replacement bar or a protein shake.

Pros: The meal frequency of this program is irrelevant for most of the days, and many people get gravitated to this.

[104]

During the feeding period, you can actually have whenever you want to. Most of the people feel that it is easier to break the feeding period into three meals, as we are already used to having three meals a day.

Cons: In spite of the flexibility of when to eat, Leangains has particular guidelines for the food you eat, especially if you work out. If you're working out, you need to schedule your meals around workouts along with a strict nutrition plan, and some people find it difficult to stick to.

2. Eat Stop Eat

Started by: Brad Pilon

Best suited for: People with healthy eating habits looking for some extra boost.

How It Works: This is my third expects you to fast for a complete 24 hours for one or two days in a week. The creator of this method, Brad Pilon, prefers to call it as "24 breaks from eating". During these 24 hours, no food should be consumed. You can actually have beverages that a calorie-free. Brad Pilon suggests to "act like you didn't fast" after completing the 24-hour fasting and go back to your normal eating habits. He says "some people need to complete the 24-hour fast during their regular mail time by having a large meal, while it is OK for others to end their fast by having an afternoon snack. You can actually time it the way you want, and as the schedule changes, you should adjust your timings.

What is the reason for this? By following this method, you are basically reducing your calorie intake in total, without actually limiting what you eat but by limiting how often you eat. If your goal is to improve your body composition or to lose weight, the regular workout sessions, resistance training, in particular, will help you to a great extent.

Pros: The program is flexible for people who think that fasting for 24 hours straight is a long time to stay without food. You need not start your diet by going all-or-nothing during the beginning. For your first day, fast as long as possible and you should increase the fasting phase gradually over time. By doing so, your body will gradually adjust to the fasting. Brad Pilon suggest that you start your fast on days where there are no eating obligations (like family lunch or work lunch) and when you are busy.

Another perk for this method is that you can have anything you like without counting calories. Nothing is a "forbidden food" for this. You don't have to restrict or weigh your food. All these factors make it slightly easier for people to follow. Pilon says, "You still have to eat like a grown-up." This method says that you can have anything you want, but it doesn't say that you can have as much as you want. Having one or two slices of pizza is okay but not the whole pizza.

Cons: Some people might find it too difficult to fast for straight 24 hours, without having any calories. It is a struggle for many people too fast for extended periods of time without having any food. Some people face side effects like fatigue, headaches or feeling anxious or cranky. But not to worry, these effects diminish over time. Some people get tempted to binge after a long fasting. This can be fixed, though it requires a lot of self-control and not all people have it.

3. The Warrior Diet

Started by: Ori Hofmekler

Best suited for: This is well suited for devoted people following rules.

How It Works: The Warriors Diet method instructs you to fast for the whole day and expects you to have a single large meal once a day, usually at night after about 20 hours of fasting. Our species are basically **nocturnal eaters**, who are inherently programmed for eating at night. The idea behind this method is based on giving the required nutrients to the body in sync with the circadian rhythms and nocturnal eating.

The main focus of the Warrior Diet fasting phase is about "under eating." you can have a few servings of veggies or raw fruits, few servings of protein and fresh juice, during your 20 hour fast, if desired. Doing this will maximize the "fight or flight" response of the Sympathetic Nervous System, intended for stimulating fat burning, boosting energy and promoting alertness. The 4-hour eating window at night referred as "overeating" phase by Hofmekler will help the abilities of the parasympathetic nervous system. These abilities include relaxation and digestion, promoting calm and aiding the body to recuperate. This will also help your body to utilize the consumed nutrients for growth and repair. According to Hofmekler, this might also help your body to burn the fat during the fasting time and in producing hormones. The order in which you have specific food groups during the four hours matters. Hofmekler suggests that you start with veggies first, then protein and finally fat. You can have some carbohydrates if you still feel hungry after having those groups.

Pros: Many people are attracted to this method as this diet allows them to have a few snacks during the fasting time. Having small snack during the day will actually make things easy to get through. People practicing this method reported fat loss and increased levels of energy.

Cons: Though it is nice to have some snacks rather than fasting for 20 straight hours, it is hard to follow the guidelines for the food that is to be taken (and when to take it), for a long term. For some people this is my third can be tricky as the strict meal plan and schedule of this method might interfere with their social gatherings. On top of that, having just one meal during the night, while following the mentioned guidelines on what two and when to eat, can actually be tough, especially for people who don't prefer having large meals at late hours of the day.

4. Fat Loss Forever

Started by: Dan Go and John Romaniello

Best suited for: This process is best for people having irregular gym days.

How It Works: You're not totally satisfied with the above listed IF diets, this is the one for you. This is a combined plan with the best parts from the Leangains, The Warrior Diet, and The Eat Stop Eat. You also get to have whatever you like on one day each week, which is a good thing for many. This will be followed by fasting for the next 36 hours, which most people may not like. After these two, the remaining time from the seven-day cycle will be split among different fasting protocols.

Dan Go and John Romaniello suggest that you save the longer fasts for days when you will be busy so that you can stay focused on being productive rather than focusing on your hunger. The training programs of this method will help the participants in losing the maximum fat with simple ways.

Pros: According to Dan Go and John Romaniello, while others are fasting every day, most of us do it regularly and with it, reaping the rewards will be harder. The Fat Loss Forever consists of a 7-day fasting schedule, which basically makes the body get used to the timetable, achieving the most from the fasting sessions.

Cons: On the other hand, if you cannot have a healthy diet during the cheat days, the Fat Loss Forever method might not be the one for you. The schedule of this method is pretty specific, and the schedule for fasting and feeding differs from day today, making it confusing to follow. You can actually note how to exercise and fast each day on the calendar for making things easier.

5. UpDayDownDay Diet (aka Alternate-Day Fasting or The Alternate-Day Diet)

Started by: James Johnson, M.D.

Best suited for: This is for disciplined dieters who have specific goal weight.

How It Works: This is an easy one. One day, eat very less and on the next, eat like normal. Take about 20% of your regular calorie intake on the low-calorie days. And so using 2500 calories or 2000 calories for men and women respectively, on the low-calorie day, the intake should be around 500 and 400 calories respectively. There are several tools online, which will help you in figuring the calories to consume during "fasting" (or "down").

For making the low-calorie days easier to stick to, experts recommend using meal replacement shakes, as they contain the essential nutrients. Rather than taking small meals, the meal replacement shakes can be taken throughout the day. Only for the first two weeks, the meal replacement shakes are to be taken, and after those two weeks, you should start having real food on the low-calorie days. Eat like normal on the next today and repeat the process. It may hard to work out in the gym on the low-calorie days for people working out daily. It is better to leave the sweaty sessions on your "fasting" days so that you don't feel exhausted. It is smart to save your heavy workouts for your regular days.

Pros: This method mainly focuses on weight loss. You can consider this if losing weight is your main goal. People who can cut the calories by 20% to 30% on average can see a weight loss of about 2 1/2 pounds a week.

Cons: People find it easy to binge on regular days, as this method is easy to implement. You need to stay on track, and the best way to do it is by planning your meals in advance so that you don't end up at a buffet or at a drive-through, taking extra calories.

Chapter 5: Intermittent Fasting Diet, Workout Regimen and the Ketogenic Diet

One of the most popular methods of intermittent fasting is the Leangains program, which has been discussed already. Here is how a typical intermittent fasting diet looks like:

- Have two meals per day
- Take a gap of eight hours between your meals.
- Work out for a few times every week and see that you exercise during the fasting window between your meals.
- On the day of your exercise, see that your diet includes meals consisting of meat (proteins), boiled vegetables and carbohydrates.
- See that you will have your largest meal of the day only after working out.
- On normal days when you don't work out, see that your diet includes meals consisting of meat, vegetables, and fats.
- Stay away from processed foods as much as you can. If it's not possible, see that the food is minimally processed. Taking supplements is of not much use either.

Thus, intermittent fasting doesn't mean you just need to have two meals per day and sleep on the couch during the remaining time. That's not how it works. You need to combine it with proper diet and workout regimen to see the best results.

Workout regimen

Heavy Weight Training

During intermittent fasting, the best form of workout one needs to employ is heavy weight training. When your body undergoes heavy weight training, chemical compounds called catecholamines are released in excess. These chemical compounds work by driving the body to release fats, particularly from the midsection, so as to burn them during the workout. When combined with intermittent fasting, heavy weight training produces best results in burning up the stubborn fat stored in places like the abdomen. Thus, it is advised that you choose to undergo heavy weight training few times a week, instead of sticking to cardio.

Walking

Another important activity that produces best intermittent fasting results when combined with heavy weight training is walking. Walking is not as intense as cardio or heavy weight training and usually, requires longer durations. The advantage of performing low-intensity activities like walking is that fatty acids stored in the body are selectively utilized for fuelling up the activity.

Lose Fat Fast by Combining Ketogenic Diet with Intermittent Fasting

Children suffering from epilepsy are advised to follow a diet rich in fats, low in carbohydrates and adequate in proteins. This type of diet is called 'ketogenic diet.' When high amounts of fat are consumed, with a low intake of carbohydrates, the body will start burning up fats instead of carbohydrates.

Ketone bodies

In general, our body converts the carbohydrates present in the food we take into glucose. This glucose is essential for the proper functioning of the brain. But, if we go on a low-carbohydrate diet, our fats get converted into fatty acids and chemical substances called ketone bodies by the liver. These ketone bodies are then transported to the brain, where glucose gets replaced by them as the source of energy for the brain. Ketosis is a state in which the blood consists of an increased number of such ketone bodies. Such increase in the number of ketone bodies will help in reducing the occurrences of epileptic seizures.

When such ketogenic diet is combined with intermittent fasting, the results obtained will astound you mainly because of two reasons:

- **Fat is burnt to a maximum extent**

As mentioned earlier, the body is said to be in ketosis if the blood has a high amount of ketone bodies. In such a state, body fat acts as the primary fuel for energy. When the body is subjected to intermittent fasting in such a state, the fat reserves get used up instantly. In such a case, burning of fat takes place much more efficiently.

- **Fat is burnt for a longer duration**

In people following the Keto intermittent diet, the levels of glucose are very less, and hence the body can enter into a state of fasting very quickly and easily. Since the state of fasting can be achieved pretty quickly, there will be more time for the burning of fats. The burning of fat for longer durations result in the quicker loss of weight.

Thus, when combined with a ketogenic diet, intermittent fasting results in the faster burning of fat, which in turn results in faster loss of weight.

Chapter 6: Health vs. Fitness

Why do people follow diets and vigorous exercise regimens in the first place? Is it to be healthy? Or is it to be fit? Even though some people use these two terms synonymously, there is a difference between health and fitness. Let us suppose you see a body builder who looks unnaturally muscular with muscles bulging up his triceps. How do you see him? You might think he looks physically fit, but does he look healthy to you?

A body builder who looks big and strong sure is fit, but is he healthy? It is a known fact that you need to be fit if you want to be healthy. But, it is possible for a person to be physically fit and still be unhealthy. For example, when you look at the pictures of certain bodybuilders, it becomes apparent to you that they have taken steroids to build their bodies. They may look strong, but we can't say if they can perform physical activities like running, jumping, or undergo a vigorous workout regimen, which are all the signs of a physically fit individual.

When you take a look at a bodybuilding magazine, you will see pictures of body builders or both genders with their muscles bulging and glistening in fake tan. You won't be able to find even a pint of fat on their perfectly fit bodies. But don't let physical appearances fool you. Those models may look extremely fit, but they might not actually be healthy. Your main goal before following any diet should be healthy and fit, and not just to appear physically fit.

Also, people think that they can eat whatever they want as long as they hit the gym twice or thrice a week. The problem is that you might achieve fitness even if your eating habits are not that great. But good health cannot be achieved through exercising or working out alone. Being healthy is more of a way of life. If you keep on eating stuff that is high in fat content or food filled with chemicals or a high percentage of preservatives, you will not be able to achieve good health even if you work out in the gym every day. It is because exercising will do nothing to reduce the damage caused by those harmful chemicals.

Also, it is true that working out promotes the overall health of an individual, but what greatly affect our health are the nutritional choices we make. We have seen many professional athletes who have battled serious health problems in their retired life. If they were so fit and athletic, what made them go through all those health problems? Ultimately, it is the nutrition and the food choices we make that decide our health and longevity.

Thus, it is important that you remember being healthy is more important than being fit; I am not suggesting that you don't have to pay attention to working out. Fitness is an important part of being healthy. It may help in the burning of fat or improve energy levels, but our well-being ultimately depends on our health and not on the size of our triceps.

Chapter 7: Should You Use Supplements?

Before you walk into a store and put the bottle of Vitamin A or C tablets in your cart, you have to stop and think about whether or not they even work for you and if they are safe or not! But, before all of that, you will need to ask yourself if you need the pills at all. There are quite a few people all over the world who have started to take these supplements – powdered form, pills or in liquid form – in order to obtain the nutrients and minerals they believe they have lost on account of the diet. You will need to remember that you do not have to take these supplements.

There are many nutritionists who have said you do not need to consume any supplements since you will be obtaining the minerals and nutrients that your body needs through the food that you consume. The other aspect to consider is that the supplements that you do consume may, in fact, cause a lot of harm to you. There are quite a few side effects to the supplements that you consume. If you have certain health issues, they may aggravate due to the supplements that you consume. It is best for you to consult a health physicist if you are bent on consuming supplements. This is to ensure that the supplements you take are integrated into the diet that you are on.

Most people have started to consume the supplements under the impression that they will be cured of any disease. This is false since no supplement has been found to cure any chronic diseases. There are times when a person will need to consume supplements in order to sustain their health – for instance, a pregnant woman will be in need of calcium during the nine months of her pregnancy since she will need to have strong bones. But, there are certain things you will need to remember. If someone says that a supplement is a natural product it does not necessarily mean that it has no chemicals in it. You will need to look at the chemical composition before you consume these supplements.

The advantage with the intermittent fasting diet is that you do not need to consume any supplements since the meals that you consume are rich in the nutrients that your body needs in order to keep you healthy. You need to ensure that you check the food that you eat in order to decide whether or not you will need supplements. If you find yourself losing out on certain nutrients, you could take the supplements for the same.

It is crucial when it comes to deciding on whether or not you will need to take dietary supplements. You will have to look at their benefits and their side effects before you choose to take one. You will need to converse with your doctor or any pharmacist in order to decide whether or not it is vital for you to take any supplements. If you do have to take any, sit with them and decide on which supplement is best for you.

Chapter 8: List of Tracking Tools

When you are on a diet, you will find it difficult to stick to the diet that you have chosen. You will probably find yourself worrying about whether or not you are healthy and if you can stick to the diet. This chapter covers the list of all the applications that you can use in order to help you stick to the diet.

Calorie Counter and Diet Tracker by MyFitnessPal

You will find that the app is ready to work the minute you install it on your phone and begin to use it. The application has a clear statistics page that will help you account for every morsel that you consume on a regular basis. You will be able to know how many calories you have consumed and will also be able to decide on the weight that you have to lose. You will find that the app is easy to move through. It has the easiest functions and is of great quality. There are a lot of people who have said that the application is a great way to change the way you eat.

Amwell

This application is great for those who are skeptical about starting a new diet. The application allows you to converse with numerous medical professionals in order to have all your questions answered. You will be able to share your medical history and will be able to gain the best advice from professionals and dieticians. You will find the interface easy to use and of excellent quality. A person who is not tech – savvy will find the application extremely easy to use! If you are looking at using supplements during this diet, you could connect with the dieticians on this application to know what is best for you.

Fitbit

Fitbit is the best way to live healthier. The company strives to create products that would change the way a person moves in order to stay strong and healthy. The products that are available to the public are often very easy to use and do not need any extra effort to use! There are products that will help you track the number of steps you have taken and will also help you know the number of calories that you have burnt. There are some other products that would help you know your heart rate and the distance you have traveled during the day. The products help you live a very healthy life.

Diet Assistance

This application is the best way to know how far you have progressed when it comes to losing weight. The developers of the app have tried their best to help you and every other person who is trying to lose weight. You will find a great way to keep track of your weight and will also be able to plan your week and identify your grocery list. You will be able to build a clean diet plan that will help you lose weight in an orderly fashion.

There are many other applications that you could use when you are working on a new diet. These tools are a few of the tools that will aid you on your journey.

Chapter 9: How Is Skipping Breakfast Helpful?

You have always been told as a kid that you must never skip breakfast since it is one of the best meals to consume to kick start your day. You may have been told that you will be smarter in school or you may have been told that you will burn a lot of fat! But, this is the rule. Are you a person who is willing to not follow the rules and become leaner and control your hormones? Well, if you are you have come to the right place! When you start the intermittent fasting diet, you will find that you are asked to consume a heavy dinner and skip breakfast. There is a reason behind this too!

The truth is that the fact that you burn fat when you consume breakfast is not completely true. This is because of the fact that you will be able to gain more lean muscle when you skip meals! That is right, you have read it correctly. It has been found that you will build leaner muscles faster than the average human being when you skip breakfast! You could also build leaner muscle if you fast an entire day! Let me tell you why the doctrine of the calories does not make too much sense. Human beings everywhere find it difficult to cope with the amount of stress they are under due to their personal and professional lives. If this were a true fact, then people who are slightly obese would have become leaner in no time when they consume sugar-free sodas, but they are not. This is because of the fact that human beings have something called hormones! Do not be surprised when you read this since you need to remember that hormones have never been logical!

Hormones are categorized into two – catabolic and anabolic hormones. The catabolic hormones are considered the masculine hormones since they are related to aggression and breaking down of substances. The anabolic hormones are feminine hormones since they are growing and are passive. The former are often associated with the functions that are performed by the body during the day while the latter are associated with the functions that are performed by your body at night. Your body needs both hormones to function well. When you skip breakfast, you are increasing the work of your catabolic hormones and negating the functions of the anabolic hormones. When the catabolic hormones begin to function, your anabolic hormones also begin to work thereby creating leaner muscle! When you are on the intermittent fasting diet, you will find yourself growing leaner because of the very fact that you skip breakfast!

Conclusion

With this, we have come to the end of the book. The book was mainly written to educate the reader about what intermittent fasting actually is and why it works. As mentioned already, Intermittent fasting is not a diet plan that says what you need to eat, but a diet schedule that says when you have your meal and when you shouldn't.

Intermittent fasting has proved to be beneficial for people who are trying to lose weight and achieve the toned look. It has also proved to be beneficial in aiding an individual in building up muscle mass. Since men and women are different physically and physiologically, they will experience different results from intermittent training. There is not a standard intermittent fasting format you could follow eyes closed to lose weight; you need to experiment with the different formats mentioned in the book and decide on what works for you.

I am ending this book with a word of caution- if you are suffering from blood sugar related conditions like hypoglycemia or diabetes, you need to consult a medical practitioner before setting out to begin intermittent fasting.

I hope I have covered all the basics and the working mechanism of intermittent fasting. I have also explained how Ketogenic diet can be combined with intermittent fasting to achieve the best results. Before trying out one of the methods of intermittent fasting, do take the advice of your physician first.

I want to thank you for downloading this book and hope that you find it informative and helpful in your weight loss endeavor.

Happy intermittent fasting!

THANK YOU!

If you liked this book, why not leave a review on Amazon? Being an independent publisher on the ever-growing eBook market, every review you post helps us reach more people and provides us with important feedback to better serve you and other readers in the future.

Also, don't forget to join the Lean Stone Book Club. It's the best way to stay up-to-date with all our books, activities and promotions. Furthermore, you'll get various opportunities to contribute to our book club (and even get rewarded for it).

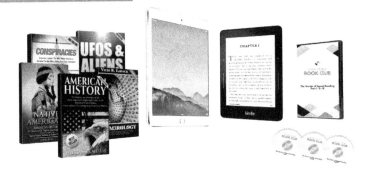

>> leanstonebookclub.com/join <<

Thank you once again for reading our book! All our kudos go to you!

LEAN STONE BOOK CLUB

CPSIA information can be obtained
at www.ICGtesting.com
Printed in the USA
BVHW041615180422
634616BV00009B/772